Gems of Costume Jewelry

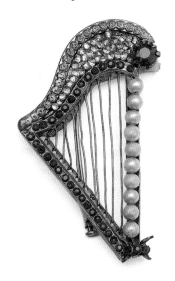

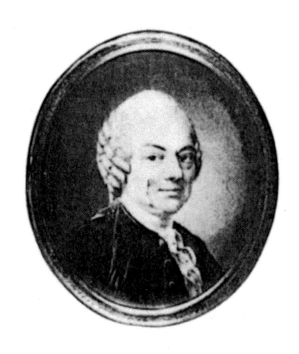

Contemporary portrait of Georges Frédéric Stras, 1785, still in possession of the family in Paris

Gabriele Greindl

GEMS OF COSTUME JEWELRY

With an Introduction by Dominica Volkert

Translated from the German by Laura Lindgren

Abbeville Press • Publishers
New York • London • Paris

Jacket illustrations
FRONT: black-and-white photograph courtesy of the Kobal Collection, London
BACK: black-and-white photograph courtesy of the Kobal Collection, London

INTERIOR DESIGN: Cristian Diener
JACKET AND TYPE DESIGN: Patricia Fabricant
PHOTOGRAPHY: Sophie-Renate Gnamm and Raoul Manuel Schnell

First edition

Library of Congress Cataloging-in-Publication Data

Greindl, Gabriele.
[Strass. English]
Gems of costume jewelry / Gabriele Greindl ; with an introduction
by Dominica Volkert ; translated from the German by Laura Lindgren.
p.   cm.
Translation of: Strass.
Includes bibliographical references and index.
ISBN 1-55859-207-5
1. Costume jewelry.   I. Title.
NK4890.C67G7413   1991
391′.7 — dc20   91-13827
                                                                    CIP

Contents

Foreword

*R*hinestones — as long as jewelry is made with this small, sparkling, man-made stone, opinions about it will vary. For many, especially for today's young generation, glittering rhinestone jewelry has become a standard accessory; for others it remains cursed, stigmatized as an imitation, a "fake." The initial motivation for the production of rhinestone jewelry was the desire to create a perfect imitation of "real" diamonds. At the close of the eighteenth century in Paris, Georges Frédéric Stras first fastened the striking imitation diamonds he had made onto silver shoe buckles and collars, and the flawlessness of his imitation soon brought him immense success.

One of the most important goals of this book is to free rhinestone jewelry from its persistent description as "fake." But where is the line to be drawn? The genuineness of a stone — whether glass or diamond — no longer suffices to define the artistry or originality of jewelry. An antique piece of rhinestone jewelry, such as a marvelous Art Deco brooch, clearly has much more artistic character than any of the many diamond pins produced by the thousands today.

Frequently, so-called genuine jewelry is mass-produced in stereotypical designs that tend to destroy the special character of the materials used. The classical "fake," by contrast, has become rare and has taken on a genuineness all its own arising from its uniqueness and the originality of its design. Furthermore, written and unwritten laws regulating the wearing of jewelry have all long been abolished. The sumptuary laws of the Middle Ages and the Renaissance lost their meaning in the radical changes brought about by the industrial and political revolutions.

The renaissance of rhinestone jewelry during and after both world wars can be explained in part by the effect dramatic social changes have had on fashion. As class distinctions blurred and divisions in society grew increasingly permeable, the difference between genuine and ungenuine jewelry became irrelevant. The twenties saw an immense boom for the rhinestone: Art Deco brooches, animal brooches, bracelets, and extravagant necklaces were commonplace. The rule was anything goes. In the seventies rhinestones became the jewelry of fashion in the truest sense: denim and velvet jackets, evening gowns, purses, and tops were all covered with the sparkling, colorful stones. Fashion — which of course includes jewelry — always reflects the static or changing nature of its time. And so it is that the unusual rhinestone pieces that grace the pages of this book not only lead to an aesthetic experience (unexpected, perhaps, for many), but also occasion a little of the social and cultural history of Europe and North America. The jewelry made by the great designers, such as Eisenberg, Weiss, Coro, and Trifari — and now rightly called classic — reveals much about the people who love this jewelry and about the environment in which it was created.

Gabriele Greindl

Rhinestones: The Cultural History of an Imitation

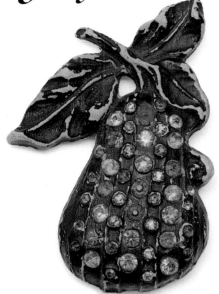

Very rare brooch of colored rhinestones set in wood, 1925

*R*hinestones — the diminutive glass stones that simulate precious gems — are today, as they have been for centuries, an accessory without which fashion would be unimaginable. This shimmering showstopper has been affixed directly onto clothes, both haute couture and ready-to-wear, as individual pieces and in elaborate compositions; it adorns belts, pocketbooks, shoes, barrettes. Its primary domain, however, is costume jewelry. Here, too, it gleams not only as a solitary stone but, best of all, in diverse combinations on the widest variety of jewelry items. The spectrum of people using it runs the gamut from renowned jewelry designers and jewelers to manufacturers of cheap baubles.

Popular and multipurpose, the rhinestone today flourishes independent of social status or class. Fascination with its visual brilliance cuts across all lines. The very fact that it is included in fine jewelry indicates a revaluation of this glass paste as a legitimate material not merely pretending to be something else but possessing a high intrinsic value of its own. Similarly, other "ungenuine" components, from man-made materials such as plastics (Bakelite, acrylic) to natural products (wood, cork), have entered into the realm of fine jewelry.

What's more, jewelry art has even drawn upon the effect of costume jewelry encrusted with imitation stones to generate new ideas for designs employing genuine materials. Indeed, in the late eighties the fashion trade celebrated a "comeback of jewelry," emulating lavishly endowed imitation jewelry. As the Düsseldorf jewelry designer Georg Hornemann put it, his collection is intended to be seen as "totally crazy, almost like costume jewelry, but genuine." The gap between art and artifice is narrowing more than ever with the materials in use today. When jewels and precious metals begin to imitate their own imitations, it would seem the line separating the "genuine" from the "fake" has been erased.

There can be no doubt that in its original eighteenth-century form the rhinestone was intended to imitate transparent precious gems, particularly the diamond. Even at that time master jewelers were happy to deal in the production, manufacture, and sale of artificial gems. Innovative grinding and setting techniques appropriate for the new materials were developed, which meant an improvement in precious-gem manufacturing in general. Even among the highest ranks of the nobility rhinestone jewelry was greatly esteemed and had its own uses. In France around 1775 Monsieur Granchez, jeweler to Marie Antoinette, advertised "en pierres de Stras d'Angleterre" (in stones of strass [rhinestone] from England); in mid-eighteenth-century England the court jewelers George Wickes and Samuel Nethertone offered a "Variety of False-stone Work"; and the Dresden court jeweler Christian Neuber's exhibition at the Leipzig Fair of 1786 featured "women's jewelry in the newest style with rhinestones and all colors of stones," which was especially well received.

In spite of their costly production, the imitation stones were sold at prices considerably lower than real precious gems, and the market for them grew very quickly. This contributed to an appreciable change in the function of jewelry. Before the eighteenth century, jewelry as a symbol of status had to a large extent been limited to the court and its ceremony, but gradually it became available to the general public, where it gained footing as a mere decorative ornament. Concurrently, there was a decline in the superstition and folklore surrounding jewelry, which maintained that gemstones possessed holy and protective powers.

Tapping the middle class as its new market, rhinestone jewelry escaped the sociopolitical disorder of the French Revolution and enjoyed active popularity throughout the nineteenth century. Industrialization made it possible at last not only for the rhinestone but for entire pieces of jewelry to be manufactured by machine. Costume jewelry became — as it has remained in the industrialized countries in particular during the twentieth century — a phenomenon of the masses.

The Rhinestone: What Is It?

The rhinestone today has come to mean artificial stone made of glass similar in color and cut to the diamond. The "fire" of a cut diamond, which makes it so fascinating and appealing to imitate, is derived from its ability to refract white light in the color spectrum. The strength of this quality is measured with a light refraction index. Ordinary glass has, for example, a light refraction far lower (1.5) than the diamond (2.42). To approximate the color dispersion of the diamond, the cut-glass stone must be foliated. The "brilliance" of a diamond or a transparent precious gem depends on its cut. The surface of the precious gem is divided either entirely or partially into facets. The angle of the facets to one another, the proportion of the top and the bottom portions (crowns and culets) of the stone affect its reflection of light. The more ideal the proportioning of the width to the depth, the greater the brilliance of the diamond. Although the rhinestone, particularly in its modern form, fails to achieve the diamond's grade of color dispersion and brilliance, its sparkle is no less spectacular, and this, of course, is what makes it so popular.

In hardness the rhinestone is no match for real stones, but this in no way diminishes its gleam. According to the hardness scale set up by the German mineralogist Friedrich Mohs, minerals are classified according to ten levels of hardness. Rhinestone has a hardness of five at most, while the diamond, the hardest substance, is at ten. With the help of a simple hardness test it is easy to tell whether a stone is genuine or merely made of glass: the colorless topaz, beryl, and sapphire, but above all the diamond, will scratch window glass, whereas glass stones cannot.

The rhinestone's characterization as "colorless glass," "diamond cut," and "diamond color" can be historically differentiated, because in this imitation stone's two-hundred-fifty-year history, attitudes toward all three of these criteria have changed. Moreover, *rhinestone* isn't the only term for the little glass stone; it possessed a number of other names as well: simulation, strass, flint glass, Mainz flux, glass flux, paste, falsestone, brilliant, diamanté, *pierres de Stras*, *pierres fausses*, and so on were, and still are, used as synonyms.

In Anglo-American areas *rhinestone* or *diamanté* has become more commonly used than the term popular before the turn of the century, *paste*, while in German-speaking countries *simili* and *strass* serve as generic terms. The term *rhinestone—Rheinkiesel* in German—has become the trade name for the cut-glass jewelry stone, although strictly speaking it refers to a material other than the diamond imitation: rock crystal. Originally this was the name given to pebbles of rock crystal, found in the Rhine River, that had drifted downstream, becoming rounded off in transit. When cut and set they have a luster similar to glass. In the eighteenth century these small stones were a favorite variation of the imitation precious gem. The Spanish and Portuguese even preferred rock crystal to glass for their imitations. And in England rock crystal took the additional name of *Bristol stone*, or *Bristow*, after the well-known mining region, whereas in France it became known as *pierres du Rhin* or *pierres d'Alençon*.

The French term *pierres de Stras* (stones of Stras) refers to the Parisian master goldsmith and court jeweler Georges Frédéric Stras (1701–1773), who experimented extensively with glass and specialized in the production of artificial stones to imitate diamonds. Due to his efforts the imitation grew closer than ever to the original. The spelling of the German term *strass* is based on mere orthographic convention. Early in the eighteenth century the German words *straz* or *strasz* were used to differentiate the glass stones from the jeweler's personal name; likewise, in French the word *strass* was in use. But as is evident from its numerous and varied names, the material known in English as rhinestone, strass, or paste was not the original invention of Georges Frédéric Stras, even if to some extent he has prevailed eponymously. Indeed, the rhinestone was a collective achievement in European handicraft that began in the seventeenth century, continued through the eighteenth century, and blossomed with improvements by Stras, but not solely by him.

Contributing to the heightened interest in diamonds was the further development and perfection in the second half of the seventeenth century of new methods for cutting precious gems. The variety of cuts, such as the Mazarin cut, rose cut, step cut, baguette cut, pear-shaped cut, marquise, briolette, and so on, was expanded sometime around 1700 with the invention of the brilliant cut by Italian stonecutter Vincenzo Peruzzi. Divided into a minimum of fifty-seven facets, this cut features an octagonal "table" with pavilion facets pointing downward and converging at the culet. With slight modifications, this is still the most frequently used cut. The wide variety of new cuts applied to imitation stones as well, and the brilliant cut created an exceptionally strong light refraction. The American term *brilliant*, which refers not only to "genuine" diamonds but to any imitation stone employing the brilliant cut, suggests that at least to some extent the qualities of sparkle and luster are more highly valued than the actual market value of the gems. Before the means existed to produce glass stones by machine, implements and tools identical to those used for diamonds were used to cut and polish imitation stones.

In addition to jewelers and goldsmiths, glasswork centers showed an interest in the production of "glass notions," that is, buttons, beads, and jewelry stones made of paste. In the eighteenth century an independent branch of the craft in Gablonz, a town in northern Bohemia, was able from the outset to specialize in imitation and glass jewelry. Wherever centers of jewelry manufacturing appeared, glass—especially in the form of cut-glass stones—was to be found. Its varied grades could all be used and it was virtually limitless in quantity. As early as the nineteenth century the German jewelry centers of Schwäbisch Gmünd, Pforzheim, and Hanau, as well as Idar-Oberstein, made use of *articles de Bohème*, Bohemian glass notions, as did French jewelry manufacturers.

In addition to its superior potential for variety in form and cut, glass offered another appealing characteristic for being processed into jewelry: its wide spectrum of colors. Jewelry made of colored glass is known to have existed since the third century B.C. in Egypt and in eastern Mesopotamia. Glass paste, composed of a mixture of sand and soda twice heated, gained luminescent color with the addition of metallic oxide and was, in all likelihood, intended to imitate various precious stones. Of course, these glass compounds were filled with numerous air bubbles, a clear giveaway of imitation stones and a problem that continued to trouble even eighteenth-century manufacturers. Artificial glass production saw its first breakthrough at the turn of the fourteenth century in Venice with the development of colorless molten glass (*cristallo*) and was crucially influenced at the end of the seventeenth century by the discovery of clear flint glass and, most important, lead crystal. Experimental procedures always involved assembling the three essential components of glass—silica, alkali, and a stabilizer—to achieve a molten glass that met the highest requirements for hardness, proper surface tension, and crystallization. The same requirements that apply to flat and hollow glassware—mirrors, bottles, drinking glasses, and vases—apply to glass stones as well, because in order to be processed further into jewelry pieces they, too, must be colorfast, hard, and suitable for cutting and polishing.

The terms *paste* and *glass flux*, concepts fundamental to the glassworker, refer to the combining of individual components in glass production. *Flint glass* and *Mainz flux* refer to special kinds of molten glass that contain lead oxide as a stabilizer.

The production of uniform, clean, colorless glass without discoloration or the necessity of redyeing requires as great a knowledge of precise glassmaking formulas as does the production of colored glass, in which it is generally necessary to decide whether to add coloration during the melting process or to dye the finished product.

Experimentation with colorless glass to create imitation precious gems began in the eighteenth century because of the diamond's high value and allure,

qualities it has possessed throughout history. But all fashion trends are subject to change, and aesthetic attitudes toward the colorless stone have fluctuated with the times, too. For example, German jewelry producers at the turn of the twentieth century tended to turn away from diamonds in spite of their value; consequently, colorless imitation stones fell from their position as the paragon of fashion.

However, glass was still used either to imitate transparent colored semiprecious stones or as a substitute for transparent colored precious stones. Cut into facets to produce, like their white counterparts, a sparkling, high refraction of light, these colorful imitations are also known as rhinestones. Following the American boom in production of rhinestone jewelry, from the 1920s on these imitations have been used in every color and form imaginable.

The Art of the Copy: Counterfeit or Imitation?

The diamond's reigning position in the hierarchy of precious gems has provided perpetual motivation for imitation. In antiquity and far into the Middle Ages healing powers were ascribed to them, such as the ability to neutralize poison, to dissolve gall-bladder and kidney stones, and to prevent epileptic fits. Supernatural effects were expected from a diamond worn on the left arm; it was believed that one was thus protected from witches' spells and from the evil eye. Deriving its name from the Greek *adamas* ("the infertile"), the diamond is recognized as a symbol of love and strength. As a birthstone it belongs to the month of April and it is said that it will impart courage and loyalty to those born in that month.

During the Enlightenment with its emphasis on rationalism, the practice of ascribing supernatural meaning to diamonds ended: at the beginning of the eighteenth century Johann Heinrich Zedler in his great *Universallexikon* (Universal Encyclopedia) denounced the alleged medicinal properties of the diamond, and in 1754 the matter was definitively settled in an article in the *Encyclopédie* by Denis Diderot and Jean le Rond d'Alembert. Even so, the diamond retained its high esteem—along with the ruby, the emerald, and the sapphire—as one of the four "water-clear" precious gems and as the hardest of all minerals. And in terms of craft and aesthetic value it ranked first in its class of colorless, water-white gems.

Techniques for imitating this stone are every bit as old as the admiration for the original. In the first century A.D., Pliny the Elder mentioned Indian methods of producing simulated precious gems in his *Historia Naturalis*. The dyeing of crystals — above all, beryl — the mixing of pastes from glassmaking materials or honey, and the use of other substances similar in appearance to polished magnetite are only a few of the many possibilities. Why these early "fake" versions of diamonds were considered to have special powers remains unexplained and today seems rather incredible.

Of utmost importance to the imitation, even in antiquity, was the outward appearance of genuineness. And this demand prevailed in the following centuries as well. Official ordinances forbidding the production of artificial precious gems — such as the edict of 1331 against the French goldsmiths' guild or the law of the Venetian Council of Ten in 1487 for the prevention of precious gem imitations — were unable to stop experimentation with the widest variety of imitations. Criminal records show that punishment ranged from flogging to banishment, even for those who had merely set imitation stones into jewelry pieces.

Well into the fifteenth century throughout Europe imitation was regarded as outright counterfeiting and was punished as willful deceit and as a violation of the law. Sumptuary laws had been laid down not only to govern individual classes of society in matters of clothing but to restrict the wearing of jewelry as well. Only the royal family, persons of nobility, and the clergy were allowed to wear gold, silver, precious gems, or pearls, all of which symbolized power and high social standing. To imitate jewels or to trade in such imitations was tantamount to a double offense against social convention: it enabled those not entitled by class or position to wear jewelry and, because the imitation stones pretended to be something they were not, they brought into question the validity of genuine stones as a symbol of the power of their wearer.

Of course, the specific association between jewelry and nobility could survive only as long as the hierarchical societal distinctions were rigidly fixed, and the acquisition of precious gems and precious metals was possible only for the upper class. With shifts in the social and economic importance of society's classes, political power and economic power were no longer inextricably linked, and the character of jewelry changed, too. It began to represent the affluence of prosperous citizens as well as high secular or clerical rank. It is impossible to pinpoint the exact date of this upheaval; rather, it was the result of a gradual process that had already manifested changes in the populace's self-image during the late Middle Ages. Eloquent testimony of this transformation is provided in contemporaneous portrait paintings depicting common people bedecked in chains, rings, earrings, and brooches.

As the circle of people for whom jewelry was a virtual ready-made accessory expanded, taboos and sanctions against imitation gemstones were removed. Imitation per se was no longer a punishable offense, unless there was proof positive of an intention to deceive. In treatises about the goldsmith's art there appeared chapters on production of simulations and formulas for the removal or application of color in stones to imitate other stones. One such publication is Benvenuto Cellini's renowned *Due trattati dell' oreficeria e della scultura*, 1568. It contains a long discourse on how, and with what materials, less valuable stones can be treated to make them appear more expensive, techniques for coloring diamonds to enhance their sparkle, and complicated formulas for the removal of color from sapphires or topaz to create imitation diamonds.

The creation of imitations and copies gained increasing legitimacy as an artistic activity requiring skillful handiwork as well as mineralogical knowledge and imagination. Even scientists began to examine precious gems not only for their chemical construction, classification, and physical properties but also for their imitability. Anselmus Boetius de Boodt of Holland, once personal physician to Holy Roman Emperor Rudolf II, published, in 1644 in French and in 1647 in Latin — which at the time was the language of science — a history of stones and jewels, including a chapter on imitations and their characteristics. This early scientific treatise was later expanded with descriptions of how to foliate stones and set them into jewelry pieces, enabling subsequent jewelers and goldsmiths to use de Boodt's book as a reference work. The French version, characteristically enough, was titled *Le Parfait joaillier* (The Perfect Jeweler).

It is glass, which could be created only through artful and complex formulas, that provides evidence of this climate of experimentation. As early as 1612 Antonio Neri had gathered together a collection of formulas, *Arte vetraria*, which was translated and revised many times, by Christoph Merret in England, for example, and in 1679 by Johann Kunckel, director of the world-renowned glassworks of Pfaueninsel in the Havel River between Potsdam and Berlin. His *Ars Vitraria Experimentalis: or, The Complete Glassmaker's Art* remained an important source of information on glass production well into the nineteenth century. He described fully the methods by which crystal, with the addition of brimstone, could be brought to burn and then quenched in water to produce a pure, diamondlike stone.

In the 1650s in Paris, at the former monastery of the Knights Templar, the first factory to produce imitation stones in great numbers was established. Under the direction of George d'Arce, crystals were produced to be sold—once they had been dyed or foliated—as fake diamonds, emeralds, topaz, and rubies. The *diamants du Temple* were the height of fashionable imitation jewelry stones for many years, even though they were also subject to sharp criticism: of only a mat brilliance, they were easily recognizable by their whitish surface and could at best be used for nothing more than theater costumes. Yet, in spite of this negative judgment, sales of the popular *diamants du Temple* were so great that Monsieur d'Arce came into a considerable fortune.

This universal fondness for glittering precious gems—even if only imitation—was to witness an ironic twist of fate when almost 140 years later, in the very place where imitation gem production had begun to develop in the seventeenth century, Marie Antoinette, a ruler who had won the antipathy of the French people, not least of all because of her fascination for costly jewels, was arrested. In 1792 the frivolous and pleasure-seeking wife of Louis XVI was consigned, along with the entire royal family, to d'Arce's Temple, which had been converted by the Revolutionary guard into a prison. Hatred of the extravagant court had recently been inflamed by, among other things, the notorious Affair of the Diamond Necklace, the intrigue to which the queen fell victim in 1785. Marie Antoinette was purported to have been prepared to pay two million livres for a necklace of 564 diamonds, twenty-four of which were the size of hazelnuts and six of which were pear-shaped and even larger. The entire story had in fact been contrived by an adventuress calling herself the comtesse de La Motte, who wanted to obtain for herself the lavish jewelry that had originally been commissioned from the Parisian jewelers Boehmer and Bassenge for Madame Du Barry, the mistress of Louis XV. "As soon as we have the treasure in our hands we will make use of it," Johann Wolfgang von Goethe had the marquise say in *Der Grosskophta*, his

comedy about the Affair of the Diamond Necklace. "We will break it up, you will then go to England and sell it, having cleverly switched it with the little stones." The drama involved one of the biggest jewelry heists ever, for which its instigator, the comtesse de La Motte, was flogged, branded, and sentenced to life imprisonment. After two years in jail, however, she managed to flee to London, where, along with her husband, she lived extravagantly on the proceeds of the sale of the stolen gems.

The temptation to commit such criminal offenses, particularly after expensive jewelry became more widely available, occasioned yet another use of imitation stones, one that is still relevant today. To prevent valuable and priceless pieces of jewelry from being stolen, copies of them were made of glass stones. The visual effect of such copies was by no means less than that of the original, nor was the pleasure of adorning oneself with these jewels, but there was no great risk to run in the event of a loss. The valuable stone locked away in the safe became, in essence, a capital asset, financial insurance in times of uncertainty. The imitation stone, which only pretended to be rare and valuable, fulfilled the jewel's superficial duty to attract attention and admiration. Even expensive crown jewels were sometimes replaced with imitations, either to prevent them from being mislaid or so that individual precious gems could be used elsewhere without disassembling the entire piece of jewelry. So it was, for example, that over the centuries the famous diamonds of the French crown jewels, the 136.75-karat "Regent" and the 54-karat "Sancy," were transferred from one piece of jewelry to another and often had to be replaced by paste copies.

The Neugablonz glass jewelry industry in Kaufbeuren has specialized in, among other things, copying select or irreplaceable precious gems. The crown of the German Reich is one of its renowned achievements. These copies of rare jewels also had a significant effect on the democratization of jewelry, once the exclusive privilege of nobility. The duplication of unique items enabled individual pieces—originally worn only by a single chosen person and admired only by a select few—to be displayed to a wide public in exhibitions and even in more than one place at a time. Every single reproduction required impeccable craftsmanship to achieve a visual effect identical to the original.

The tragic consequences that can result from a good imitation are vividly described in Guy de Maupassant's sentimental, allegedly true story "La

Parure" (The Necklace). The wife of a lowly civil servant borrows a wealthy friend's diamond necklace to wear to a social event hosted by the town minister. It so happens that by the end of the evening's festivities the necklace has disappeared. In order to buy a comparable replacement, the couple must spend all their meager savings, and they are forced to move into a shabby attic apartment and go deeply into debt. From that point on their life is one of sacrifice and poverty. It is not until ten years have passed that, ashamed of their past carelessness, they tell the friend who had loaned them the jewelry of their true circumstances, only to find out that the lost necklace was a mere imitation and worth no more than a few hundred francs.

Such mix-ups depend on cheap or cheaper components having the exclusive mission of pretending to be their valuable counterparts, which means, of course, that they must deny their own natural character. A "strict" copy of expensive jewelry traditionally purports to look exactly the same as the original jewelry supposedly did at one time, and subsequent glass imitations model themselves after this copy. However, once imitations had become acceptable in high society, paste stones were permitted their own identity to a certain degree and were no longer something to be ashamed of. Original glass jewelry designs were created and the rhinestone came to be regarded less as an imitation than as its own jewelry type.

The gap between the value of the copy and that of the original is, as is true of fashion in general, subject to the dictates of a period's taste. The rhinestone alternated between phases of functioning purely as an imitation and phases in which it asserted its independence. There have also been times when it fulfilled both functions simultaneously, as is the case today. As a mere imitation without intrinsic worth the rhinestone sometimes depreciated in value, yet it was at the same time praised as a fascinating, glittering material offering exciting new possibilities.

The Close of the Seventeenth Century: The Onset of the Art of Imitation in England

*I*n 1676 Englishman George Ravenscroft (1618–1682) succeeded in bringing about a fundamental improvement in glass production. His invention of lead crystal meant great progress in the development of colorless glass. His formula for the combination of raw materials was crucial to his success, as is always the case with the production of paste. As a technician at the Savoy Glass House in London, Ravenscroft developed his mixture partly to compete with the Venetian glass arts industry and partly to find a substitute material for the wood ash that had been used up to that point. His mixture consisted of pure white sand, potash, saltpeter, and minium. The latter material determined, depending on how much was used, the lead oxide content, which in turn affected the luster, colorlessness, and light refraction of the final product.

Ravenscroft was of course not the first to use these exact ingredients; traces of lead oxide appear even in the various glasses of antiquity, as well as in more modern formulas, such as those in Antonio Neri's *Arte Vetraria* of 1612. And some reports maintained that the actual formula was created by an Italian, a clear indication that the influence of Venice is not to be underestimated. What is certain, however, is that Ravenscroft's achievements included, among other things, the discovery of a stable, balanced ratio of individual ingredients, and that his influence on glass production in general was crucial. The London trade, under the patronage of no less a figure than the duke of Buckingham, was the first to produce lead crystal on a large scale. Thus lead-glass stones became available for jewelry-making and were celebrated well into the eighteenth century as "English paste," cut and set into silver.

Two properties of lead crystal, however, subsequently presented extreme difficulties. Even when the raw materials used were very pure, the compound had a tendency to discolor, usually turning yellow. Bismuth, thallium, or other bleaching substances were added to combat what was considered a deterioration in quality. Moreover, because of the high lead content, the end result was not especially hard; in some cases the glass failed even to reach the hardness of grade five. A high refractive index was possible only at the expense of reduced hardness. Furthermore, the mixture had to be heated very precisely to keep the number of air pockets to a minimum.

But it is precisely these difficulties in glass production at the time that enable the collector today to recognize imitations at a glance. Besides air bubbles in the stone, the facet edges may have lost their sharpness and the polished surfaces may have become dull. Chemical changes in the glass substance can cause a filmy cloudiness to set in and streak the interior. When the original fire of a stone containing lead has thus been lost, it is immediately identifiable as an imitation stone of historical interest.

The Surrogate Becomes Fashion: Pinchbeck and Colleagues

As great as the advances in the field of glass production and in the acquisition of popular and affordable costume jewelry were, imitation precious gems were not all that was needed to bring jewelry to a wider audience.

Especially effective was a discovery made by the English watchmaker Christopher Pinchbeck (1670[?]–1732). By fusing 128 parts copper, 7 parts brass, and 7 parts zinc, he succeeded in producing a dark gold-colored alloy that suffered little oxidation and could be used as a substitute for gold. This mixture subsequently became known simply as pinchbeck. After Pinchbeck died, his son carried on the business, trying to keep the exact formula for the alloy secret. Of course, he was unable to prevent the copper-and-brass alloy from being recognized and it was soon duplicated; after all, it was feverishly sought after by jewelry producers and jewelry wearers alike as a substitute for the expensive precious metal gold. In Paris there soon appeared a comparable metal compound by the name of *pomponne*, commemorating the place where it had been produced — the Hôtel Pomponne in the rue de la Verrierie. In Lille a man named Rentz discovered yet another copper alloy, the so-called *semilor* or *similor*; the Parisian Leblanc

named his special mixture *métal Leblanc*; and in Mannheim, Germany, an alloy of 7 parts copper, 3 parts brass, and 1.5 parts tin known as Mannheim gold was created. Still another compound was tombac (from the Malay *těmbaga*, meaning copper), which ultimately played a central role in the production of costume jewelry.

All these alloys have in common a gold hue that tends to range between red gold and yellow gold, depending on the content of zinc. *Semilor* and *pomponne* usually require supplementary gold coloring. The high copper content of these substitute products made them especially pliable; for instance, tombac, when finely hammered, can serve as imitation gold leaf, which was originally called talmi. (Today the meaning of talmi covers much more ground, and essentially all such surrogates and imitations are often labeled as talmi.)

Paper-thin foils of metal were directly involved in the jeweler's art, particularly in the setting of transparent stones. Since the Middle Ages stones, especially cut stones, have been set in gold, silver, and copper in order to intensify their play of color. Through complex processes, and depending on the length of time they were heated, layers of metal would take on different hues. Although these methods met with rather varied opinion over the years — excitement grew in the meanwhile over the imitation of natural gem colors — they were quite common even into the nineteenth century, and foliation is still a common method of enhancing the brilliance of rhinestone jewelry today. Pinchbeck, *semilor*, and tombac were important not only for foils but most of all for settings, because they allowed cheaper stones to be inexpensively placed into jewelry pieces. While these alloys originated in the seventeenth century, they did not experience their first full blossoming until the nineteenth century, when the colored precious gem — or rather, its imitation — again entered the limelight. The reason gold-colored settings were seldom employed in the late seventeenth century and throughout the eighteenth is that colored stones played only a minor role during this time. The gold substitute nevertheless became a popular material for other jewelry pieces, which largely dispensed with precious stones even at the time of the diamond's zenith. It was used for watchcases and chatelaines — decorative plaques worn on the belt or waistband from which were suspended, on chains, clocks, medallions, signets, and even dainty miniature books.

The Eighteenth Century:
The Rhinestone Reaches New Heights in France

The eighteenth century was the last century in which the court set fashion trends to any substantial degree. But the status of the court was to shine one last time, rich in ideas and imagination before it became definitively controversial in this field. This was especially true of centrally governed France where the French Revolution came to a dismal and ruthless end. During the reign of Philippe II of Orléans (1715–1723), Louis XV (1723–1774), and Louis XVI (1774–1792), the stylized art of fashion rose to mannered affectation: the pannier skirt became bigger and bigger (a circumference of up to approximately eight feet meant one could pass through doorways only by stepping sideways); the décolletage ever more plunging; bows, ruffles, and festoon ornamentation more luxurious; headdresses and hairstyles more ostentatious. The fabric used most was silk, which, in contrast to the material used during the reign of the "Sun King," Louis XIV, was lighter, more flowing and airy, and predominantly of soft-hued and pastel colors. Men's clothing, too, was more graceful, refined, and lighter than in the past century. Court clothing was distinguished by richly ornamented, full-cut jackets, jabots and sleeves generously endowed with lace, and knee breeches profusely decorated with bands or buttons. Although the prestige of such fashion remained unchanged, the image that the court now presented was new. The ostentatious and pompously theatrical baroque was superseded during the rococo period by an affectedly whimsical conduct no less "unnatural." Central to this playful attitude was the demonstration of *bon ton* or *bon goût*, which members of the court felt was important both to adhere to and to enrich with many innovations. Various concepts of chivalry and eroticism offered opportunities to show proof of a wealth of ideas. And this was directly reflected in fashion, which fell subject to the art of suggestion. Women's skirts were shortened, and beneath the bouncing hemline the shoe or even the foot up to the ankle was visible; specially fastened draping ribbons or artificial flowers, which reached their peak in popularity at this time, signaled amorous messages, depending on how they were worn: at the neckline, around the neck, or in the hair. One of the most well-known examples was a bow poised at the front of the décolletage, suggestively called *postillon d'amour*.

It is no surprise that in this environment the brilliant diamond was to triumph and become the focus of jewelry items. Its setting, once a dominant focal point, was increasingly subjugated to the role of the mere mounting. The predominant use of silver encouraged this development, since it emphasized the fire and refractive quality of the colorless stone without introducing a new color. For this reason, especially pure and high-quality jewels were set *à jour*, that is, open above and below to expose the stone to the greatest possible amount of light. The closed setting, by comparison, permitted foliation, which enabled less valuable stones or glass to display a greater shine. This method of setting engendered still another technique, which had no equal in the gleam that resulted: the *en pavé* setting. In this type of setting the stones were abutted like paving stones to create the appearance of a continuous surface of countless facets. Under the candlelight of the chandelier, which multifariously refracts light in its glass prisms, the shimmer and radiance of this fashion was amplified all the more. It is not surprising that the imitation stone found acceptance in a period that delighted in illusion and superficial effects.

Artificial baubles, which were not limited in form and method to jewelry made with stones, partly transformed the traditional and partly created the new. The Sévigné brooch, designed by Gilles Légaré, one of Paris's most famous seventeenth-century jewelers, was especially well received. The Sévigné brooch consisted of a double bow from which dangling pendants were suspended or to which stones were fastened. Of similar construction was the girandole, a design used not only for brooches but also for earrings and necklaces with pendants. The bow could be replaced by a cross-shaped element, but the number of pendants was limited to three, with the middle one hanging somewhat lower than the other two to create a drop-shape outline. Another type of brooch was the agrafe, a hook-and-loop fastening worn either at the décolletage or on the shoulder and favored in those days to secure nosegays and floral sprays in plumes or bunches. The aigrette, predecessor of the diadem, took the same motif. Worn in the hair, usually to one side, it often contained springs so that individual blossoms or panicles would be set into motion with the slightest movement of the head. This popular technique, which was perfected at this time, was termed *en tremblant*.

Just as versatile were the different versions of necklaces. Bands of fabric, velvet, or precious gems were worn *en carcan*, that is, close to the neck, with a girandole, a pendeloque-cut stone, or a solitaire fastened to the front. There were also chains that hung down into the neckline with an additional central pendant plunging deep into the décolletage. The pendant could usually be detached and used as a brooch. The rivière necklace came into fashion, its large, individually set stones often surrounded by smaller ones attached with petite links. Sometimes many rows of festoons and other pendants complemented the dominant stones, forming an expansive glittering mesh. The necklace of the notorious Affair of the Diamond Necklace is alleged to have been of this type.

The preference for wearing several pieces of jewelry at the same time necessitated coordination of the different pieces. Thus complementary sets or, in the language of the trade, parures were created. The "classic" parure consists minimally of a necklace and earrings, but it may also include brooches, bracelets, aigrettes, and the like. If the set lacks a necklace, it is called a demi-parure.

Of particular importance in men's fashion, though not exclusive to it, were shoe buckles and decorative buttons, which also welcomed the ornamentation of precious gems. The shape and size of shoe buckles changed frequently and quickly; sometimes they were large, sometimes small, sometimes round, oval, quadrangular, or square. There was apparently no limit to the imagination where shoe buckles were concerned, and yet in an instant they became unfashionable. As a symbol of royal taste, which lavishly decorated shoes seemed to exemplify especially well, buckles were out of fashion by the end of the century and were forced to yield to laces, which the lower classes had long been using to secure their footwear.

From the Goldsmiths' Guild to the Union of the Imitation Gem Manufacturers

In eighteenth-century France and elsewhere, guilds were more or less of the same order as those established in the Middle Ages. Guilds (in French, *corps* or *corporations*) were alliances formed by craftspeople or tradespeople to regulate both the practice of their trade and its economic conditions according to joint rule. The guilds were recognized by the governments in power at the time, which, in conjunction with the top guild representatives, made sure that the statutes were obeyed. On the one hand, guilds enabled their members, as much as was possible, to work undisturbed by other workers or dealers; they helped members to obtain benefits and represented the members' individual interests. But on the other hand, these associations had strict and strongly regulated committees that threatened stiff sanctions and prosecution if the statutes were not upheld.

During the ancien régime in France, goldsmiths were organized into *corps des orfèvres*, whose statutes essentially went back to the ordinances of the fourteenth century. Two groups of craftspeople could count themselves as goldsmiths: the *orfèvres-bijoutiers*, who worked primarily with precious metals to create tableware or so-called fancy goods, including watchcases, knobs for canes, buttons, buckles, and the like, and the *orfèvres-joailliers* (or simply *joailliers*), who were jewelers in a stricter sense, that is, they were manufacturers of jewelry pieces that featured, as was fashionable at the time, the gemstone. In addition to production and handling, goldsmiths were allowed to sell their wares, whereas a simple *marchand* — a dealer — was allowed only to market his wares but not to produce or process them.

The grinding of diamonds and their imitations was reserved for the lapidaries, who employed grinding wheels of their own design along with a line of simple tools for manual grinding. The cut stones were subsequently mounted by *metteurs en œuvre* into assigned settings prepared by goldsmiths and silversmiths. The polishing of the finished jewelry was done by *polisseuses*, or polishers.

Every single operation of the jewelry trade, from the production of individual pieces to the marketing of the final product, was painstakingly separated from all other operations. Only a master guild member could acquire the right to engage in the complete process. This strict division of labor — or, rather, the limitation on the number of people allowed to practice all operations — made for an organization that could be closely observed. It eventually became the standard for the guilds producing the most precious and valuable materials.

To achieve the title of master, a formal course of education was required, which included a period of study and years of service as a journeyman, usually combined with a period of travel. Prerequisites included independent social status, legitimate birth, and a good reputation. School terms ended with an examination in which one had to prove his knowledge and readiness; of central importance was one's prentice piece, or masterwork.

The statutes of the French goldsmiths' guild stipulated the completion of one's twentieth year as the minimum age for the *maîtrise*, the master's exam. To become eligible for the *maîtrise*, one first had to complete the journeyman's exam, which was usually followed by a period of time spent traveling. Guild regulations limited the number of masters' positions, so it was not always easy to find a firm where one could assume such a position after the final exam, be it through marriage or testamentarily arranged succession. Under a strictly regulated employment contract, an otherwise fully valid employee who had not completed the *maîtrise* could work in a firm as the *compagnon*, or head journeyman.

Through an overabundance of regulations the guilds were able to maintain their internal hierarchical structure over a long period of time and, since they were powerful and large associations, their influence on social and political life throughout Europe was not to be underestimated. But this very rigorous organization of production and trade also hindered the flexibility and responsiveness of the economic system. New markets and businesses spelled danger for the guilds; the so-called unguilded were effectively excluded from the market, and in a competition that was therefore unequal, attempts were made to forbid them from practicing their craft. After lengthy and complicated transformations the guild system was eventually supplanted by the principle of free enterprise.

In France free trade was introduced as a direct result of the French Revolution in 1791. This momentous legal decree was certainly not unexpected. In the course of the eighteenth century new regulations relaxing the strict guild rules had arisen, clearing the way for the legislation of 1791. As guilds became increasingly limited, decisive steps were taken toward new production and trade methods.

With self-confidence among the non-nobility increasing, fashion sensibility changed, as did attitudes toward the art of jewelry. The growing demand for jewelry — which was an important factor in the emergence of imitation jewelry — was just one of many indications of this new self-confidence. Technical innovations and advanced knowledge of chemistry and physics lent additional support to this process and brought about the first upward trend in imitation production in general. By the 1830s, guild regulations had already relaxed to the point of dying out, thus making it possible for genuine and imitation precious stones to be combined in a single piece of jewelry. This was a significant change for the traditional statutes, the primary function of which was the observance of the rule that only precious gems and precious metals were to be handled by guild members.

To control the steadily growing demand for imitations, on July 27, 1767, the French government approved the foundation of the guild of imitation gem makers, the *joailliers faussetiers*, which soon had a membership of over three hundred. The privilege to produce and distribute jewelry, which entailed carrying the burden of meeting requirements of exclusivity, was taken from the *corps des joailliers*, and all guild statutes were affected in even more drastic ways. To begin with, the limitation of the title of master to a set number was done away with, as was the requirement to complete a masterwork. Anyone who considered himself in a position to become a master and who believed he was able to command an atelier and produce simulated jewelry was eligible to do so. The elite master jeweler, who had to earn his title not only on the basis of ability but also through considerable expenditure of time and finances, suddenly found himself surrounded by colleagues who, if they possessed a talent for the craft and a business sense, met with success much faster.

With these transformations, new working methods for the manufacture of imitations were also developed, because the ungenuine stone was no longer considered a mere imitation but was acknowledged to possess an intrinsic value. For example, the lower hardness grade of glass proved felicitous for creating new styles of cut. It was thus possible to create, for instance, the so-called *calibré* cut, in which a stone is cut to the exact same shape as its setting, filling it completely and leaving no space or gaps in between. Especially with square shoe buckles, which became stylish over the course of the eighteenth century, this technique of setting was used to achieve a sparkle even into the corners.

The multivolume *Encyclopédie* by Diderot and d'Alembert of 1765 listed five cuts for the *diamant de Stras* that differed from the typical diamond cuts of the time. With their somewhat asymmetrically arranged facets they were still further removed from the original model of the "genuine" stone. These so-called fantasy cuts remain a popular feature of imitation stones today. And other specific methods of foliation for imitations were developed: with an amalgamation of tin foil and quicksilver a mirrorlike reflection could be created to simulate a high refractive index in the paste stone.

Despite all the new techniques of jewelry production the traditional art of the goldsmith still persisted, except that now it was forced to grapple with phenomenal competition. This competition created the basis for differentiation between exclusive, unique pieces and mass-produced wares, and it only intensified over time.

The man whose name was originally bestowed upon what is now less commonly known in the United States as strass and more frequently referred to as the rhinestone lived during these times of transformation. As a goldsmith he increased production of imitations, contributing significantly to the relaxing of rigid guild ordinances.

Georges Frédéric Stras

So many anecdotes and fantastic stories have circulated about the inventor of strass that it is little wonder that he has occasionally been regarded as a mere fabrication himself. However, historically verifiable information about the life of Georges Frédéric Stras, though not abundant, proves that he did indeed exist.

It is certain that Georges Frédéric was born on May 29, 1701, in Wolfisheim, a village not far from Strasbourg, and that he was the youngest of seven children of the minister Jean Frédéric Stras and Marie Marguerite Stras, née Redslob. His mother was from Eckartsweier in Baden; that is why both French and German were spoken in the immediate family, as was true throughout Alsace, the greater part of which was granted to France at the end of the seventeenth century.

In 1714, at the age of thirteen, Stras became an apprentice to Strasbourg goldsmith Abraham Spach,

under whom numerous German jewelers completed their education. Five years later, on June 13, 1719, he completed his apprenticeship. What sort of journeyman's piece he completed is no longer known.

The next fourteen years of Stras's career and whereabouts are unclear. Most likely he traveled, perhaps to Germany. His language skills and his connections with German colleagues in Strasbourg lend credence to this theory.

In any event, in 1733 Stras found himself in Paris, working as the *compagnon* of a Madame Prévost, who was running the jewelry workshop of her deceased husband. After earning his master title that same year, Stras went independent and opened an atelier on the Quai des Orfèvres on the Ile de la Cité. Although his masterwork is no longer extant, the hallmark that Stras's *maîtrise* entitled him to stamp on his jewelry pieces is known: it bore his initials, G.F.S., and a crowned sword; next to it was the mark of the city of Paris. Like all hallmarks, it was registered with the Paris assay office. As "Maître Orfèvre et Joaillier privilégié du Roi" (master goldsmith and jeweler bestowed with privileges from the king), Stras began his career, which brought him both great esteem and a handsome fortune. He worked on the Quai des Orfèvres for almost forty years, until his death on December 22, 1773, at age seventy-two. What distinguishes Georges Frédéric Stras is not the claim that it was he who invented the brilliant little paste stones but the fact that he seems to have been the first goldsmith and jeweler to perfect the existing techniques of imitation with glass paste that had been tested in many places, developing further methods in the process, and most notably, handling imitations with great style.

In him, artisan and practitioner were united; theoretical considerations were skillfully combined with the talents of a businessman who presented fine products for men and women. He was so successful that his surname became a recognized trade name that endured for the next two centuries. Even today the word *strass* can be found in many encyclopedias, and in Germany it is a household word (even if most are unaware of its actual origin).

No other producer of imitations achieved the same level of success, not the clever Monsieur d'Arce, nor Christopher Pinchbeck with his metal alloys, nor George Ravenscroft, who produced lead glass.

In 1740, when Stras was only thirty-nine, *strass* first appeared as an entry in the *Dictionnaire de l'Académie française*, where it was described as a substance used for the imitation of diamonds and named after its inventor. No other information on the inventor — his first name, profession, or place of work — is given, indicating that even at this early date strass had become a material concept; the person Stras was considered to be of mere etymological interest. Thirty years later the *Dictionnaire portatif de commerce* listed strass as a stone named after the person who had first sold it in great quantity — Stras found mention as a dealer, not as a producer.

Georges Frédéric Stras regarded himself primarily as a tradition-conscious goldsmith and jewelry dealer who not only produced finished jewelry pieces but also produced and traded in individual parts, offering them for sale to be further processed, whether by other jewelers or setters.

This characterization is evident from his business and calling card, which was designed and produced in 1735 by Charles Nicolas Cochin — exactly one year after the founding of his own atelier. Richly decorated with leaf and tendril work, putti, a sea deity, and a maiden spilling the contents of a cornucopia as a symbol of wealth and abundance, the card read: "Stras — royal jeweler and jewelry dealer, resident of Paris, Quai des Orfèvres, House 'Duc de Bourgogne' — hereby announces to the honorable setters of precious gems in all countries, provinces, and nations, that he is in possession of the secret of producing in finished form foils in silver and all other colors. He skillfully colors all kinds of stones to resemble those of the Orient. He sells superior gold powder and fulfills orders for diamonds and other precious gems, processed or unprocessed, in greater or lesser quantities. All at very reasonable prices."

Above all Stras advertised his abilities in the coloring and foliation of jewels. These two methods brought an enriched, intensified look to the gems, a look that was the taste in those days. Silver or colored foils, such as gold powder, when placed beneath the precious gem in the setting, increased the stone's radiance, and a light stain supported and beautified the stone's natural hue. An example of ideal brilliance and hardness was the *pierre d'Orient* (stone of the Orient); one of the highest priorities of the jeweler was to simulate this model of perfection by artifice, such as by the use of colors and foils. Stras did not advertise his substitute materials or rhinestones. Whether this omission indicates that he was not pursuing the production and sale of the paste diamond at this time or that his intention as a newly established master goldsmith was first to announce and prove his traditional

craftsmanship remains unknown. Some thirty years later, however, Georges Frédéric Stras had achieved such great success from the production of paste diamonds that he produced and sold imitation jewelry exclusively.

So reported Stras's colleague Pouget the Younger in his jeweler's handbook *Traité des pierres précieuses* (1762). Pouget also mentioned a goldsmith by the name of Cheron who had so thoroughly devoted himself to the imitation diamond that in time the term *cheron* came to refer to a false precious gem. Cheron varied the formula for lead crystal to achieve a harder product. The hardness and the resistance of the glass stone were the central concerns of all creators of imitation stones.

"Je travaille tous les jours à la dureté" (I am constantly at work on the hardness), Stras allegedly remarked. He finally triumphed over Cheron in this area, apparently, because his competition faded away and the term *cheron* likewise disappeared from fashion consciousness. Exactly why this happened is impossible to say, because only the ingredients (white sand, alkali salt, minium, lead oxide, and saltpeter) but not the exact quantities or ratios of each or the length of heating time were handed down. Perhaps it was Stras's business acumen alone that brought him such sweeping success. His commercial connections extended throughout France and even to England and Holland.

The offer Stras announced in his 1735 business card to all "Messieurs les Metteurs en œuvre de tout Pays, Provinces et Nations" was often taken up over the ensuing decades. His estate included many bills of sale made out to the most renowned jewelers and gem setters of the time.

In the second half of the century imitation jewelry became extraordinarily popular as an item of fashion that did not balk at the sumptuous and extravagant models of the French court. Madame Pompadour and her successor Madame Du Barry purchased articles from Georges Frédéric Stras, and Marie Antoinette herself was supplied with paste jewelry ordered by court jeweler Granchez. Granchez's business, Au Petit Dunkerque on Quai de Conti, was one of the top sources of elegant jewelry innovations and remained so until 1835.

The preference of women of the court for real jewelry is well known, but they were also interested in imitations, as is clear from the high regard that paste gems acquired in their time. Rhinestones not only provided cheaper jewelry for the less well-to-do, but they also fascinated the entire fashion world, regardless of social stature or name.

Bestowed with royal privileges, the jeweler and goldsmith Stras catered to the general populace but considered himself to be of equal status with the *joailliers de la couronne* — the court jewelers. And Stras had yet another claim to the status of a court-commissioned goldsmith: his niece Susanne Elisabeth, who came from Strasbourg to stay with her uncle in 1750, married Georg Michael Bapst, the nephew of Jean Melchior Bapst, who had been established as a goldsmith in Paris since 1725. Georg Michael was named *compagnon* and successor to Stras, who was unmarried and childless; Bapst died, however, in 1770. His son, Georges Frédéric, Stras's grand-nephew and godson, took over his father's position and, after 1789, the directorship of his great-uncle's atelier. Trained by court jeweler Jacquemin, he also took over the position of court jeweler, following in the same tradition as the Bohemian who had become the victim of the intrigue in the Affair of the Diamond Necklace. The famous Maison Bapst, which in following years was frequently assigned to reset the crown jewels and which existed until 1930, had in Georges Frédéric Stras's heir one of its first champions.

Joseph Strasser: Vienna's Claim to the Parisian Rhinestone

Not only in French dictionaries and encyclopedias of the eighteenth century, such as those mentioned above, is Stras clearly identified as a French goldsmith born in Alsace, but in German publications as well. Johann Karl Gottfried Jacobsson's *Technological Dictionary*, published in Berlin and Stettin, contains an entry for "Strasz," which states that the "Straszburger Jeweler" was "superbly talented."

So it is all the more surprising that early in the nineteenth century the legend of a certain Joseph Strasser from Vienna arose. Even today this legend obstinately continues in a wide variety of publications on jewelry, fashion, and handicrafts. Amusing as the stories about Strasser may be, they differ in a crucial way from the stories about the Parisian Stras: they cannot be substantiated, and positive biographical data on Joseph Strasser is nonexistent. There is no birth certificate, no death certificate, there are no business documents, no pictures — in short, nothing

to allay the suspicion that Strasser is purely a product of the imagination.

In the world of fashion Vienna was by no means insignificant. At the end of the seventeenth century schools for the fashion trade were already being built and became highly regarded. With the Congress of Vienna in 1814–15, Viennese fashion was able to make an international name for itself. Still, Vienna always saw itself as outdone by Paris, whose preeminence the Austrian city was never quite able to attain or completely overtake. And if Viennese women's styles were occasionally acknowledged to be of "a more attractive nature" than the "newest French apparel," as Friedrich Nicolai stated in his 1784 *Description of a Trip Through Germany and Switzerland*, the fashion of Vienna, particularly in the eighteenth century, still stood in the shadow of *couture Parisienne*.

Given this situation, it is no wonder that an attempt might have been made by Viennese jewelers to take credit for the splash rhinestones had created in the fashion world and thereby gain the advantage over their Parisian rivals. This supposition is not all that farfetched, nor is it completely untrue, considering that Georges Frédéric Stras was neither the sole nor the patented inventor of the rhinestone. Since the early eighteenth century, cut-glass gems had been produced in other areas as well, such as the north Bohemian glassworks of Seidenschwanz, Turnau, and Gablonz. And these Bohemian glass notions were sold in markets in Vienna.

The originator of the story of Joseph Strasser is unknown. But the anecdotes about him should not be ignored; although untrue, they constitute part of the rhinestone's sparkling history.

Constant von Wurzbach's account of the case of Strasser in his 1879 *Biographical Encyclopedia of the Empire of Austria* is especially vivid. Even though he admits that "history, anecdotes, and rumors become mixed," he describes, without being able to produce any exact data, a jeweler and Viennese citizen Joseph Strasser, who had a "street-level" store in Josephstadt. Interested in chemical experimentation, Strasser produced myriad colored glass pastes and displayed the successful results in his shop window. One day he mixed green flint, iron oxide, alumina, sodium bicarbonate, and limestone, creating a pure, colorless mass that, when cut and polished, imitated the diamond perfectly. He set these paste stones into luxurious pieces of jewelry and asked his wife and daughter to test the reaction to his new product. The moment was opportune, as a ball was soon to be held in a hall at the Viennese New Market. The Strasser ladies appeared at the ball in full bejeweled splendor. The jewelry aroused such tremendous awe and wonder that the proud Joseph Strasser was immediately arrested because, it was believed, such astonishing jewels could only have been stolen! After a torturous night in jail the inventor was finally able to convince the authorities that the diamonds were only imitation jewels.

The incident did not pass unnoticed by the royal family. Kaiser Franz Stephan, who studied precious gems and was deeply interested in experimentation with diamonds himself, invited Strasser to court for a demonstration of the paste formula. In one version of this story, Empress Maria Theresa advised the townspeople of Josephstadt to sell the invention in Paris, where one increasingly encountered such innovations. She even paid Strasser a handsome sum to make his start abroad easier. In another version, the empress remains much more distant: remembering the 1732 decree of her father, Karl VI, forbidding the "common people" to wear jewelry, she allegedly prohibited Strasser from continuing production of his imitation gems. Disappointed by the empress's class conceit, Strasser left Vienna and went to Paris, where he sold his formula to a Frenchman. Subsequently called *pierres de Stras* — garbling the name of the inventor — the Viennese brilliants reappeared in their rightful birthplace, now credited with being a Parisian creation, as the patriotic and contentious Wurzbach angrily observed.

This incident was combined with another that further inflated Strasser's abilities and indicated that others had taken advantage of his invention in order to reap the glory for posterity. It is said that the famous British optician John Dollond came to Strasser's Josephstadt shop on the very day when Strasser was sitting in jail. Having spotted a piece of green flint glass in the shop window, Dollond was curious about its composition and structure. But because of the owner's absence he had to make do by asking the daughter, with whom he immediately fell in love. At the ensuing wedding, Strasser gave his son-in-law the paste, a mixture of flint glass and crown glass. And in 1757 Dollond used this very mixture to construct his achromatic lens. By combining dispersion and convex lenses of flint glass and crown glass respectively, Dollond created a compound lens that was practically free from prismatic colors.

In this case, as with many other anecdotes about rhinestones, it is relatively safe to say the story is a mere fabrication. No evidence of a marriage to a Viennese woman is given in the biography of Dollond, who developed the achromatic lens in 1757 together with his son.

Both of these stories did, however, find their way into Viennese popular literature and magazines, and they met with great success on the stage in plays that of course have since slipped into complete obscurity. In 1858 the comedy *Pierres de Stras* by Salmoser (actually, Adolph Schmiedl) opened, and the anonymous novel *The Fake Diamonds*, which told the love story between Dollond and Strasser's daughter, was serialized in a newspaper but never completed. A little less than a hundred years later, in 1940, a story called "The Diamonds of Vienna" was set to music in an operetta by Kurt von Lessen and Alexander Steinbrecher. Sham, kitsch, legends, and fantastic traditions are so inextricably entwined in the history of the rhinestone that it is tempting to attribute the mysterious glass paste composition to a conglomeration of myths.

The Nineteenth Century:
European Rhinestones Enter Mass Production

*B*y the beginning of the nineteenth century the bourgeoisie had thrust itself into the forefront not only of society and politics but of fashion, too, and began to play a dominant role in fashion changes. The fashion magazines and women's journals that had begun to appear during the second half of the eighteenth century acquired an even greater middle-class readership. Circulation increased as fashion innovations deluged the market.

The most important prototype for these periodicals was the monthly *Mercure de France*, which first appeared in the eighteenth century and reported on the latest fashions of the court and from Paris. It also featured a section reserved for business advertisements. England's best-known fashion journals of the time were *The Lady's Magazine* (from 1770) and *The Gallery of Fashion* (1790–1882). In Germany one of the earliest publishers of such periodicals was Friedrich Justin Bertuch, who in 1786 first published with Georg Melchior Kraus *The Journal of Luxury and Fashion*, which continued until 1826. "Jewelry and bric-a-brac" had its own column, and jewelers advertised regularly in an enclosed newsletter devoted exclusively to advertisements. This magazine was subsequently imitated by countless others, among them *Fashion Gallerie*, from 1795; *General Fashion News*, from 1799; *Berlin Fashion Mirror*, from 1832; and *The Fashion World*, from 1865.

Such publications were largely responsible for the broad intensification — or rather, the very creation — of a fashion consciousness that transcended class boundaries and led from mere imitation of the establishment to the determination of specific fashions for particular classes. Political events were also directly influential, because after the French Revolution all those outside the ranks of the nobility sought to disassociate themselves from the hated aristocracy. This trend was most visibly reflected in the clothing of the time. The extremist sansculottes had rejected short breeches (*culottes*) as a matter of principle and adopted trousers instead; they wore shirts opened at the chest and the coarse-weave neckerchiefs of farmers', laborers', and seamen's garb. Expensive jewelry was naturally disapproved of; at the very most rings or medallions of nonprecious metals with en-

graved dates of important Revolutionary events or portraits of Revolutionary leaders found acceptance. This Revolutionary costuming was of course imitated outside of France — in Berlin, for instance — but it was also ridiculed and considered suspect. The desirability of such an obvious solidarity with the lower class was still debatable.

The Revolutionary costume of the Jacobins and Girondists, by contrast, experienced sweeping success and set fashion for the bourgeoisie in the following years. The men's and women's fashion concepts that had emerged in England at the end of the eighteenth century were regarded as particularly progressive and underwent a revival. Essentially, fashion turned away from the affectations for which the French court had become famous and toward a style of clothing that was regarded as natural: the full-bodied pannier disappeared, as did horsehair or oil-cloth padding, which had lent men's jackets their form. The preferred materials were no longer silks but simpler cloth like cotton or wool; colors were much more subdued. The vertical line was once again emphasized in closely cut dress coats and loosely flowing dresses. Jewelry was worn only with great reservation; men's clothes in particular dispensed with jewelry as a result of this drastic fashion change. Jewels and jewelry became almost exclusively the domain of women's fashion.

A reemerging taste for classical antiquity and enthusiasm for the republican governments of the past influenced both women's clothing — the white, high-waisted, corsetless chemise dress came into fashion at this time — and jewelry. With the crowning of Napoleon, the French court revived the tradition of extravagant ceremony, yet the presentation and decor adhered to what was now the preferred style. Although expensive materials such as silk and brocade were employed once again, it was bourgeois fashion that provided the model for the court and not the other way around. The fundamental changes in the self-confidence of the middle class were quite apparent.

The most striking innovation in nineteenth-century costume jewelry was the use of a rich variety of colors, which regained popularity. In the eighteenth century gold, rather than silver — which had a tendency to flake — had been predominantly used for the back side of diamond settings, and now it took prominence on the front side of jewelry as well. The colorless stone still held an important position, but it no longer played the leading role. Its sparkle remained as fascinating as ever, but the colorless stone found a new use as a decorative element rather than as the central feature of a jewelry piece. As chips — that is, as small, irregularly faceted stones — they might encircle colored stones, medallions, engraved gems, cameos, or imitations of the Wedgwood earthenware so popular in nostalgic fashion.

The tendency of fashion to revive the designs of historical periods did not stop at the classical. The Renaissance and the Middle Ages were also rediscovered during the nineteenth century and led to new directions in fashion with the ever more popular theme of patriotism. Imitation jewelry took on a completely new aspect, in that it could be used to imitate centuries-old patterns that had accompanied such clothing. Of course, these new creations were anything but historically accurate; new elements of style were combined with pseudoauthentic ones in a typically colorful hodgepodge that was a reflection more of contemporary taste than of the epoch being imitated.

The iron jewelry that came into vogue during the Napoleonic Wars was unabashedly patriotic. It often carried self-congratulatory political mottos, such as "I gave gold for iron" or "traded for the good of the country," intended to demonstrate the national spirit — an action that would be repeated again in later wars. One of the main centers of production of this type of jewelry was the Gleiwitzer Ironworks in Schlesien. The stylistic model for this remarkably international cast-iron jewelry was not only the French *style cathédrale*, but more than anything else, the Gothic style of England, which had already been using steel as a jewelry material since the eighteenth century. Iron jewelry enjoyed great popularity in France after Napoleon captured Berlin and confiscated the casting molds from the Prussian iron foundry and brought them to Paris.

Faceted and polished steel, produced in great style primarily in Birmingham, England, presented a serious rival to the rhinestone, because it was more economical to manufacture and its selling price was therefore lower than that of paste, especially paste set in silver. And the glittering iron oxide marcasite — often actually the highly resistant pyrite, or fool's gold — also became prominent as a fashionable imitation stone. The rhinestone, particularly the colorless variety, experienced greater difficulty maintaining its top position in fashion in this century than during the rococo era. Nevertheless, mountings of steel or other metal alloys rapidly became common, thus keeping the paste stone in constant use.

Heavy gold chains, brooches set with colored stones, and long, multisectioned earrings, whose massive designs complemented the heavy clothing materials then in fashion, experienced a revival. But perhaps the greatest revival was that of jeweled headwear. There were sticks and combs, both worn at the back of the crown of the head, and the ferronière, which had not been seen since the Renaissance. Typically, the ferronière consisted of a strand of gold or pearls that encircled the head, and from which a small pendant hung down onto the forehead. The time was right once again for the imitation bauble; since jewelry was now worn by a relatively wide circle of people, substitute materials — pinchbeck and other alloys of gold imitation, for example — became common on a large scale.

The nostalgia for national and artistic traditions naturally aroused other sentiments as well. Personal emotions, including friendship, love, and mourning, took on such significance that a profusion of items symbolically expressing these emotions were produced. Special symbolic character was attributed to the ring. Friendship rings, sweetheart rings, and mourning rings experienced a peak in popularity as did silhouette medallions, portrait lockets, and heart pendants. The marquise ring in particular acquired new esteem because its pointed oval ring plate offered enough space for sentimental displays. Priority was placed not on the manufacture of precious and expensive materials but on the depiction of personal sentiment. Popular motifs included clasped hands, eyes, knots, forget-me-nots, urns, and letters of the alphabet. The arrangement of different colored stones often held coded messages. Trinkets such as colorful "harlequin jewelry" came into fashion, and anagrams were created using the first initial of the name of each stone: for example, REGARD, from Ruby, Emerald, Garnet, Amethyst, Ruby, Diamond. Such sequences — red, green, dark red, violet, red, and white — were frequently set in paste stones, forming anagrammatic arrangements for DEAREST, SOUVENIR, PENSEZ À MOI, and similar sentiments. The name of a beloved person, the initials of the children in a family or of revered family members, signs of the zodiac, and the like were frequently arranged this way.

An especially popular element of sentimental jewelry was the lock of hair of a beloved person, which could be employed in a picture medallion or braided into chains, bracelets, or brooches. In addition to such commemorative items, sentimental jewelry also included special mourning jewelry made of jet, a strongly bituminous lignite, which when cut and polished takes on a deep velvet black tone. When dyed black, even glass could serve as a substitute. Known as French jet or Vauxhall glass, it was produced and distributed on a large scale by the British jeweler Elijah Atkins.

Not unlike these keepsakes, remembrances of jubilees, anniversaries, particular places, and historical events, often of a military nature, also appeared. Flags, fleets, and cannons were popular motifs. And the emerging desire to travel, typified by England's upper-middle-class custom of the grand tour, but also by the increasing tendency of Germans to travel as a part of their education, gave rise to a new branch of industry: the travel souvenir, which most frequently took the form of jewelry. Italy, Europe's most popular travel destination at the time, led the way in this new development.

At the same time, a wide interest in national folkloric traditions arose and was reflected in fashion. Along with a liking for the newly discovered cultures of the Mediterranean and the Near and Far East and a fascination with Byzantine and Moorish styles, national costumes and the peasant costumes of various nationalities came to be considered chic and were even socially acceptable to the court. Of course, in this case, too, authenticity left much to be desired, and more stylized pseudocostumes, such as are common even today in Germany — the dirndl, for example — were created. Jewelry based on peasant models and designs of national custom complemented the new fashion. Thus the garnet experienced an unprecedented boom (mainly in its native Bohemia) accompanied by red-colored rhinestones.

Sentimental and souvenir fashion brought a wealth of figural motifs into jewelry production. Bouquets and flower baskets, cornucopias, half-moons, stars, harps, musical instruments, and insects — most of all, butterflies — gained popularity. Colorful Vauxhall glass backed by shiny metal foils was frequently used to create shimmering wings for insects whose bodies were made of gold-colored metal alloys. The demand for realistic representation was great, and when the technique of electroplating was developed in 1836, plant or insect designs were sometimes coated with a thin layer of gold, silver, or copper. As Adalbert Stifter noted in his introduction to *Colored Stones* (1852), jewelry design began to express an appreciation for the small things in life.

For the nobility's *petite tenue*, that is, unofficial "light" dress, it was considered thoroughly fashionable to adorn oneself with such sentimental ornaments. The same style was observed in the German courts of the Biedermeier period and in the English court, where Queen Victoria, during her more than sixty-year reign, significantly contributed to the wearing of romanticized jewelry by the upper classes well into mid-century, in spite of the rapid changes that clothing styles underwent in the course of the century. But whether the fashion of the day called for a pannier or a crinoline, a simple chemise or an elaborate bustle and corsetting, whether the dress was full-length or the feet were exposed, simple and inexpensive jewelry enjoyed great popularity. And today as well, little pendants, chains, or rings worn as everyday jewelry are popular in all classes of society. If a real diamond also shines in such an ornament, it is unassuming and understated, because the rhinestone is considered both proper and adequate for such accessories.

A Second Rococo, the Theater, and the Demimonde: The Return of the Diamond and the Shine of New Baubles

Although the popularity of jewelry among the bourgeoisie began with the rejection of aristocratic pomp, jewelry remained an essential part of the royal image. This was especially blatant in France: no sooner had monarchical rule been reconsolidated than grand attire returned to play a pivotal role. And jewelry of highly precious materials, as always, symbolized power and imperial status. Once again the diamond ranked highest among the jewels employed. For the privileged it was still regarded as the most valuable precious stone. While fashion had changed in terms of jewelry designs and settings, the appeal of jewelry encrusted with diamonds remained as strong as ever. Empress Josephine, wife of Napoleon, was notorious for her predilection for luxury and was by no means less fond of jewelry and jewels than her ancien régime predecessors.

As a jewelry piece complementary to high-waisted dresses, the diadem regained popularity and, as was true earlier of the aigrette, it offered a suitable place for diamonds or their imitations, but the preference was for them to be set in gold and worn in unpowdered hair. The rich gold and gem jewelry of Empress Josephine and her ladies-in-waiting was captured in Jacques-Louis David's monumental coronation paintings of 1806, although these paintings do not reveal the fact that the empress, like her royal predecessors, gladly donned rhinestone jewelry. The attraction of the imitation survived unharmed through all the societal upheavals. The emergence of a new enthusiasm for diamonds and, naturally, for the colorless rhinestone as well, and the fascination with attractive combinations of transparent stones set in silver was characteristic of the nostalgia for the eighteenth century. It is ironic that this development started in France, where in the course of the French Revolution fashion had become unmitigatedly political and royal attire was vigorously rejected. This direct use of clothing to promote political goals had of course not lasted.

In the nineteenth century, a newly strengthened class consciousness developed among the upper classes, who reverted to the old, prerevolutionary hierarchy. Beginning with the Congress of Vienna (1814–15), continental Europe experienced the period known as the Restoration. In art history, especially in the areas of costuming and the decorative arts, this period is called the second rococo. But in terms of fashion, which had already become disengaged from direct political reaction, the second rococo did not apply until after the middle of the century. Louis Philippe, the Citizen King, contributed fundamentally to the revaluation of the eighteenth century when in the first half of the century he renovated and opened to the public the palace at Versailles, which had been so badly neglected by the Directory and the First Empire during Revolutionary times.

During France's Second Empire, a spirit of splendor in fashion emerged with Empress Eugénie, and in Austria with Empress Elisabeth—the legendary Sissi. This period was regarded as a direct throwback to the rococo, not least of all because of Eugénie's enthusiasm for Marie Antoinette. Women's fashion alone was affected: the crinoline gained popularity, as did the laced bodice; the décolletage was trimmed in lace—the so-called bertha—and light materials, such as silk and tulle, as well as flounces were revived. The patterns of the past century provided incentive for individual designs that merely conjured up history rather than reproducing it exactly and that presented a unique display of luxury and opulence surpassing the splendor of the authentic rococo. To some extent the king's court began anew to set the tone for fashion after which the haute bourgeoisie and the newly arisen moneyed aristocracy modeled itself.

In contrast to Marie Antoinette's time, however, the simpler and more modest fashion of the bourgeoisie managed to assert itself as a strong competitor. The resulting conflict, however, eventually found a resolution: each style was consigned to a particular time of day and occasion. Official appointments, society evenings, and balls required grand, luxurious attire; for daytime activities modest clothing that satisfied an increasing need for practicality was required. Even the ladies of the upper classes proved themselves to be increasingly mobile, going out of the house and engaging in sports, such as horseback riding, tennis, and skating. Thus an elaborate clothing etiquette was created that affected more than just the noble set. Nothing could make for a more glaring faux pas than the wrong attire. The fashion code, developed primarily by the upper classes, remains in effect in certain circles today, where it is considered out of place to wear an evening dress to afternoon functions or to appear in a little black dress or street clothes at gala evening society events.

For jewelry design, these distinctions bore ample fruit, because the evening toilette or ball toilette naturally demanded expensive and striking jewelry, necklaces, earrings, hair combs, or decorative hairpins. The stylish pretenses of the late eighteenth century, including the preference for colorless stones usually set in silver, was taken up along with the technique of using moving components to achieve an enhanced shimmer for cut stones. Brooches were experimented with again, using such techniques as the hidden feather, which evoked the *en tremblant* effect, or a whole strand of stones *en pampille*, like raindrops spilling down. Frequently such jewelry could be taken apart and worn as an ensemble.

The décolletage was again a point of focus. By incorporating a glittering effect into the bertha, attention was directed toward the cut of the clothing and toward the jewelry itself, which was known as *devant de corsage*. Partially bent into an S shape and hung in generous lengths up to a foot, which in turn were supplied with moving parts, these breast pins were anything but inconspicuous and intentionally emphasized the tightly corseted female bust. The traditional floral motifs of the eighteenth century — leaf and flower tendrils, bouquets, ribbons, droplets, and festoons — experienced a comeback, but now they were even more extravagant, intended to show off the wealth of the owner. The old aristocracy met with real competition from the moneyed aristocracy and haute bourgeoisie. And rhinestones as a substitute for diamonds were used by all, often on genuine mountings that frequently consisted of a combination of various precious metals. Platinum increasingly came to be the preferred metal for highly valuable jewel settings. In 1851 the chemist Wilhelm Carl Heraeus of Hanau succeeded in achieving the melting point of this metal by means of the oxyhydrogen gas blowtorch he had invented, thereby making it possible to process the metal further. Just as in the rococo period, well-known jewelers used genuine and ungenuine stones alike in the production of expensive jewelry. The finished product was always expertly crafted and the settings well finished.

One of the most famous examples of the French *devant de corsage* made of rhinestones is a brooch in the shape of a twisted vine by the award-winning, outstanding Parisian jeweler and goldsmith Alphonse Fouquet. His exquisite jewelry creations of precious metals and gems made him one of the top designers of fine jewelry in nineteenth-century France. Animal forms, so popular in sentimental jewelry, also found acceptance in more opulent jewelry: birds, insects, snakes, and lizards — studded with diamonds or rhinestones — sparkled on brooches, pendants, bracelets, and rings. Although realistically shaped, these jewelry pieces were not created with an eye toward naturalism; rather, the emphasis was on their gleam and glitter.

Shimmering, dazzling jewelry was too highly desired by ladies of lesser wealth and social standing for them to do without it entirely. Abundant and widely circulating journals and magazines contributed substantially to the establishment and spread of fashion trends. The theater also became influential, receiving wide attention on the fashion pages of magazines. Famous actresses constantly appeared in women's journals, less in praise of their artistic abilities than to show off their costumes. Contemporary boulevard plays were frequently referred to as "toilette plays" by serious critics when they presented one society scene after another and constant changes of costumes grew more important than dramatic content. On occasion, fashion houses and jewelers saw to it that the stage became a second runway to display their wares.

The wardrobe and jewelry of Zerline Gabillon Würzburg, Charlotte Wolter, Eleonora Duse, and especially Sarah Bernhardt filled fashion publications all over Europe and became the inspiration for new creations. The Viennese soubrettes Marie Geistinger and Josephine Gallmeyer lured the public into the operetta houses, the Vienna Theater, and the Josephstadt Theater with their bejeweled costumes. Of course, much of the extravagant jewelry used in the theater was made of imitation materials, even if prima donnas frequently boasted of appearing in real jewels belonging to their families. The jewelry Sarah Bernhardt wore in her countless performances all over the world was made by well-known goldsmiths such as Georges Fouquet and René Lalique, and the internationally acclaimed actress shopped in exclusive Paris stores and workshops, including Maison Gripoix and Bijoux Bardach.

As an economical substitute for the stunning, gleaming diamond, the rhinestone met with a much higher demand from the theatrical world than it had from master jewelers; consequently its market grew considerably. For many, rhinestones presented the only possibility of owning such sparkling baubles. But it was not only actresses, singers, and dancers of the small and provincial theaters who formed the new clientele; the girls and women of the lower classes also became customers. Settings became cheap, and the paste stones were not necessarily fastened with care. Of primary importance was the outward appearance, an effective first impression. Aluminum, which was first produced in 1825, was used as a new substitute for silver. The jewelry industry was only too happy to seize upon the pervasive desire for glittering jewelry.

In certain bourgeois circles enthusiasm for such jewelry soon diminished; it was found irritating and cluttered. The "fake" jewelry was regarded as tawdry and worthless theatrical baubles. This growing aversion was stirred up by a group of people not without influence in the fashion world of the time — the courtesans and other women of the so-called demimonde, whose salons fulfilled a social function despised by bourgeois convention. This conflict is treated in Alexandre Dumas fils's *La Dame aux camélias* (1848), which not only offered a starring role for Bernhardt in its stage version but was also the basis for Giuseppe Verdi's opera *La Traviata* (1853). Dumas portrayed the life of the demimonde not in disparaging terms but, rather, in contrast to the supposed morals of the bourgeoisie. Beauty, attractiveness, expensive clothes, and very visible wealth were important criteria in the world of the salon ladies. Their attempts to surpass one another knew no bounds; each competitively sought to demonstrate, for instance, the wealth and importance of the financier keeping her. It is said that there was an outright war between two Parisian rivals, Caroline Otero and Liane de Pougy, that was temporarily brought to a halt with a sensation caused by La Belle Otero. Having heard that Otero would be dining at Maxim's, Pougy appeared in full bejeweled splendor, determined to steal the show from her opponent. Otero, however, employed a different tactic: entering the restaurant without a single piece of jewelry and dressed simply in white, she was followed by a maidservant who almost collapsed under the weight of a basket brimming with jewels and jewelry. Even if the story isn't true, it is at least a charming fabrication. Similar stories of the demimonde often formed the central plot of popular theater pieces of the time.

This conglomeration of reality and appearance, theater and real life, and actual and pretended wealth, symbolized by the glassy, pretty, glistening, and yet not truly valuable jewel, found expression in a figure of speech that was on many tongues in the nineteenth century, "A false diamond is like a pretty woman without soul, morals, or ethical worth." The conservatism of the underlying concept is clear, as is the rejection of the imitation around the turn of the century by a newly emerging aesthetic chiefly involving handicrafts. Supporters of the Art Nouveau, Jugendstil, Liberty Style, Modern Style, and Arts and Crafts movements, which were sweeping Europe, were not opposed in principle to ungenuine substitute materials, such as the many colored glass pastes and copper alloys, which they eventually incorporated into their work. Much more negatively viewed was the fact that the rhinestone, already an imitation itself, had become a model for other substitutions.

Eighteenth-century-style jewelry set with gems was now regarded as traditional, outmoded, and of no interest to innovative, progressive artists. Rhinestones did appear on typical Jugendstil jewelry pieces but played only a subordinate role — similar to their use in sentimental jewelry — as mere decoration to lend a little sparkle to soft, rounded, and stylized floral forms. Although Jugendstil artists employed imitations in a manner similar to that of sentimental jewelry, they energetically opposed commemorative jewelry and sought to overcome what they considered excessive naturalism by using designs inspired by earlier Japanese art.

The demand for jewelry, however, had grown to such an extent and the diversity of trends in art was so great that limitation to a certain defined style was virtually impossible. The expansion from master jewelers to a jewelry industry had advanced considerably, and even though the skillful and artistic elite continued to create individual pieces, more and more jewelry was being mass produced.

Rhinestone and Mechanical Production: The Jewelry Industry

For the skilled trade, the most pivotal achievement of the French Revolution was the establishment of a free marketplace. It was introduced in France in 1791, in Prussia in 1810, in Austria in 1859, and in 1869, with the enactment of the law on trade regulations, in the North German Confederation, and it opened up new perspectives essential to a free-enterprise-oriented economy. Supply and demand in the handicraft fields could now be directly correlated, and new workshops were built or small ones enlarged as occasion demanded. Commercial interests began frequently to overpower concerns of craft and artistry.

One aspect of this sweeping societal change was the growing demand from all strata of society for jewelry as an expression of a bourgeois sense of self-worth. This meant effective work methods were needed just as urgently as materials that could be efficiently processed. Time was money in jewelry production. A new jewelry industry was subsequently founded, organized according to the principle of the division of labor. Existing centers of jewelry production, that is, places where goldsmiths' guilds, jewelers, or precious gem grinders were strongly represented, offered themselves as bases of operation. The alliance of these professions as well as the environment of increasingly stiff competition were influential in the relatively rapid switch in methods of manufacturing.

In Germany the establishment of factories for the production of jewelry was concentrated in areas traditionally known for gold and precious gems: Schwäbisch Gmünd, where goldsmiths had been situated since the fourteenth century; Hanau, an early-seventeenth-century retreat for French and Walloon goldsmiths; and Idar-Oberstein, since the seventeenth century the site of a well-known agate grinder.

Pforzheim's jewelry and watch industry, founded in the eighteenth century, was a predecessor of the new commercially oriented production. In 1767 Margrave Karl Friedrich von Baden had called for the founding of a "watch and fine steel factory," which was expanded just three months later to include jewelry wares. Even in that early period, work at this manufacturer was performed according to a division of labor. In 1838 Pforzheim alone had fifty-four jewelry manufacturers, by 1887 there were 453 firms, and by 1890 over ten thousand people were active in the production of jewelry, while in Hanau and Schwäbisch Gmünd there were some two thousand employees working in jewelry factories.

Crucial to the industrial revolution were the advances made in technique and in commercial art. Machines to streamline working methods were built. For example, rolling, friction, and hydraulic presses superseded the embosser and engraver. Whereas formerly the goldsmith had to lay a hand on every single item, now trained workers could quickly produce numerous and identical editions.

Electroplating, perfected by the London firm Elkinton & Co., made it possible to cast a design and produce series of jewelry pieces. Engraved ornaments were made with the help of the rose engine, which enabled uniform inscription of mounted models. Polishing machines and spool machines for work with filament were developed, as well as lathes, drilling machines, and cutting machines. From the 1830s on, such innovations were used by all jewelry manufacturers.

As these new machines entered into industrial jewelry production, the traditional standards of handicraft in the goldsmith's and jeweler's art had to be redefined. Several distinct categories precisely describing the quality of jewelry materials and processing were established.

For "fine" wares only alloys of precious metals, precious stones, and top-quality pearls could be used. They had to be produced exclusively by hand, although division of labor was allowed. "Medium-fine" wares also required precious metals, but the percentage of the precious metal in the alloy could be lower, and less valuable stones, including glass, were permitted. These wares, too, were produced by hand, but mechanical aids could also be employed. By contrast, machine production was reserved for "*courant*" or "simple" wares, of fair to middling quality, and "*doublé*" wares, which were made of less valuable gold and silver alloys, were plated with gold, silver, or other metals, and used all sorts of imitation stones as well.

The hallmark, which dated back to at least the Middle Ages in most European countries and was accompanied by special marks identifying the place, year, and master craftsperson on the object, was revived and standardized over the course of the nineteenth century.

In Europe a system of evaluation using 1,000 as the standard of purity replaced the earlier system of gauging levels of purity by the karat for gold and half-ounce for silver. The required minimum for fine jewelry wares was 333 thousandths (9 karats) for gold and 800 thousandths (13 half-ounces) for silver. In Germany after 1888, the observance of this system was regulated by a federal law whose provisions remain in effect today. For jewelry, the supplemental marks of a half-moon for silver and a sun for gold may also be used.

The terms of identification used in England since time immemorial are "Britannia," which refers to a content of 95.8 percent silver, and "sterling," which consists of 92.5 percent silver. The engraved marks used today were established in 1890: sterling silver is stamped with a lion rampant or couchant, Britannia silver with a seated figure of Britannia.

In France the Brumaire Law of 1798 assigned numerical values to gauge levels of quality: 1 indicates 950 thousandths and 2 indicates 800 thousandths of gold or silver, and 3, used only for gold, indicates 750 thousandths. Until 1809 these figures were integrated in a stamp of the Gallic cock and from 1838 in a stamp of the head of Minerva, the goddess of handicrafts and the arts. Small objects of gold were stamped with an eagle's head, and those of silver with a boar's head. For medium-fine and *courant* wares either the smaller content of precious metal is specified or their precise makeup is omitted entirely.

By contrast, silver plating or gold plating must be identified as such in most countries. Identification of ingredients in alloys containing no precious metals is not required; at most they are identified with the stamp of the manufacturer. Identifying the country of origin with the words "made in" began to appear at the turn of the century on jewelry pieces made expressly for export to England. In 1887 England demanded such identification to protect the domestic production of wares, a precautionary measure that many countries adopted in their own import regulations. Before the phrase "made in" came into common international use, a separate stamp was developed for that purpose, too. With factory-made jewelry the intention was, among other things, to tap new markets in foreign countries; consequently this stamp gained ever increasing importance.

Over the past century the German centers of jewelry production — Schwäbisch Gmünd, Pforzheim, Hanau and Idar-Oberstein — increasingly made wares in the medium-fine, *courant*, and *doublé* categories. Of course, they also produced exquisite jewelry both with precious materials and after the designs of esteemed artists and designers. Such noteworthy artists as George Kleemann, Franz Böres, and Emil Riester of the Pforzheim firm Zerrenner, as well as Christian W. Müller and Adolf Huber, were some of the most important designers. In the Jugendstil tradition they often used simple materials for their designs and favored small rhinestones.

The greatest commercial breakthrough, however, came with mass production of *courant* wares. Tombac, brass, copper, semilor, aluminum, and Alpaka (a trademarked German silver) increasingly served as materials for settings. Supplemental processes such as anodizing, sulfonation, galvanizing, and bronzing were improved by technology and used most of all with silver to achieve new color variations. Glass was used in a variety of colors and forms as a substitute for precious stones.

The real stronghold of production of *courant* and *doublé* wares and above all of the rhinestone was Gablonz in Bohemia on the Neisse River. With a tradition of glass production dating back to the sixteenth century, Gablonz developed a method of jewelry production completely different from that of the old established gold and precious gem centers with their master craftsmen. To a certain extent the Gablonz jewelry industry came about coincidentally: the abundance of water in the Iser Mountains led to the establishment of numerous grinding shops, which soon began specializing in the processing of hollow glassware. In the eighteenth century, as an offshoot of the glassworks, there arose producers of glass flux, which in turn was cut in the grinding shops. Producing glass notions of all colors, Gablonz began a busy trade, and by the end of the eighteenth century the little glass stones were no longer sold exclusively as individual pieces but in settings as well.

The glass trader Johann Schwan was the leader of this new development; in 1784 he supplied his customers for the first time with buttons made of cut-glass stones set in tin. A colony of metal handicrafts producers soon followed in his wake, creating settings for his notions, as well as a group of beltmakers who fastened the metal settings and paste stones to the final jewelry products. Characteristically enough, the number of beltmakers was much higher than the number of goldsmiths, because with the production of glass stones in Gablonz the production of "ungenuine" jewelry was a given from the very start: in 1805 there were only two goldsmiths compared to fourteen beltmakers. In 1817 Philippe Pfeiffer founded the first factory to produce earrings, pendants, signets, and rings; by 1838 the first mass-production press had been introduced.

The Gablonz industry could already boast of highly efficient operations. It possessed, in fact, an astonishing wealth of specialized tools and conveyors: the "kettlemaker," which produced settings for glass stones (with a minimum of four prongs or claws for securing each stone), the electroplater, a metal dyer, engraver, porcelain painter, stone dryer, and so on.

Differentiation between highly specialized work procedures and the division of labor among various people allowed unskilled or semiskilled workers and free-lancers to be employed, which meant, on the one hand, that family-run businesses were faced with increasing mechanization. On the other hand, a sense of community was strengthened, since the creation of a finished piece of jewelry required interdependent activity. Generation after generation of individual families were active in the jewelry trade, and workshops were passed along. The Wünsch, Rössler, and Zasche families belong to the rich tradition of Gablonz craft guilds. Even after their expulsion, in the aftermath of World War II, from Gablonz (which in the meanwhile had become part of Czechoslovakia and renamed Jablonec), and the establishment of a new colony in Neugablonz-Kaufbeuren, their working methods were long retained.

A substantial part of the industry consisted of the creation of the "imitation." Colorless, faceted paste stones were mirrored to achieve the sparkle of the rhinestone. In the first half of the century there was much experimentation with chemical compounds to produce a colorful substance that not only created a silvery, mirrorlike gleam on the visible side of the glass stone but also acted as a protective coating against the surrounding setting. Before mechanical means were invented to tone down the color of the stone's underside, this task had been done by hand — another procedure free-lance help could take care of.

The definitive breakthrough in mass production of rhinestone jewelry in Gablonz came later. In 1892 Daniel Swarovsky and Franz Weiss in nearby Reichenberg constructed a polishing machine and opened a stone-grinding factory. This technological innovation was soon introduced in Gablonz as well, so that "machine stones" were now produced. Swarovsky left for a time and created direct competition in 1895 by moving the base of his operations away from Weiss and establishing a grinding shop in Wattens in Tirol. The "Tirolean stone" sold like hotcakes, enabling Swaravosky to enlarge his factory continually. Even today the Swarovsky firm is one of the most important distributors of the finest rhinestones, and—almost a hundred years since its founding—still produces exclusive costume jewelry.

The Gablonz jewelry industry, however, was already so well established that the new Tirolean firm was unable to harm it. Imitation jewelry from Gablonz maintained its position in the world market, even if it soon met with criticism. In 1895 Adolf Lilie wrote in his *Report on the Political District of Gablonz* that "Gablonz articles" were "only for maidservants and half-cultivated people."

But from the viewpoint of aesthetics and materials such an elitist judgment could do nothing to check the rise of the glittering glass stones in cheap and simple settings. "Gablonz" or "Bohemian" articles were not only distributed to German jewelry centers for further processing, they were also ordered by French firms, such as Dalloz in Paris.

Large firms specializing in economical costume jewelry were founded in many countries in the second half of the century, as entrepreneurs experienced an increasingly bustling trade. Just as Gablonz and Swarovsky sold rhinestones and other glass stones for further handling, other factories offered individual machine-made pieces in addition to their finished jewelry pieces. Frequently, independent goldsmiths took advantage of the ring metals, ring bands, links, settings, and other prefinished parts available to them. The Parisian firm Ferré, for example, published catalogs illustrated with suggestions on how ornaments set with stones could be made from the components they produced.

The costume jewelry business had an important agent in Piel Frères, a firm located since 1855 at 31 rue Meslay in Paris. In 1880 the proprietor, Alexandre Piel, took over the presidency of the Chambre Syndical des Bijoux d'Imitation. At the world exhibition of 1889 and 1890 the firm displayed Piel's *bijoux de fantaisie* creations, which were praised by the jury for, among other things, their economical yet well-crafted quality. Schwäbisch Gmünd, Pforzheim, and Gablonz were in contact with Piel Frères and were often

inspired by Parisian designs, which they sometimes even copied. In London, new stores specializing in imitation jewelry were successful, as were firms that dealt in precious jewelry, such as Asprey & Co.; in short, more and more establishments sprang up. Notable companies included the Parisian Diamond Company and Faulkner Diamond Company, which had headquarters on distinguished Bond Street and Regent Street respectively, making them neighbors of the most well-known jewelry traders. In the face of such competition, these well-known firms eventually produced "imitation jewellery" of their own, often copying the designs of "genuine" and valuable pieces.

The same phenomenon was seen in Paris: *bijoux de fantaisie* firms and producers—for example, Alexandre Royé, Madame Navez, Besson, and Galand—began to capture the interest of fashion-conscious jewelry wearers, and established jewelers such as Cartier also designed "ungenuine" jewelry, in which cut-glass stones glittered in place of precious gems.

In 1846 Louis François Cartier had already stirred Empress Eugénie's interest in Maison Cartier, which still flourishes today. Since 1906 the Parisian firm Van Cleef & Arpels has been successful as well. Early on, both were able to extend their business worldwide and to establish branches in New York and Palm Beach, setting up boutiques for "inexpensive" jewelry as well.

Demonstrating Technological Possibilities and Perfection: Rhinestones at the Industrial and World Expositions

Although the rhinestone, like the diamond, lost popularity as a jewelry item after the French Revolution, interest in the production and processing of the imitation gem remained strong. Its complex formulas presented a tough challenge for the jeweler. At first it was scientific curiosity more than commercial interest that played the decisive role; the fashion trends at the time were moving in another direction. The 1820s and 1830s saw more and more technical interest in methods of producing glass, including lead glass compounds and rhinestones. Important experimenters were F. Bastenaire-Daudenart, Julie de Fontelle, and in particular the chemist and jeweler Douhault-Wieland, whose *Mémoire* (1820) we have to thank not only for the description of the furnaces needed for melting, but also for a precise, illustrated formula. After 1818 he put his theories into practice and produced jewelry pieces using imitations.

Such achievements in craft and technology provided a major attraction for the industrial exhibitions that had been common since the mid-eighteenth century. Branches of craftsmanship and commercial trade displayed the range and development of the national industry. Top wares were premiered. At the Exposition des Produits de l'Industrie Française of 1819 the jury awarded a prize of 1,200 francs for the best rhinestone formula in connection with the most attractive rhinestone jewelry. Douhault-Wieland outdid his toughest competitor, the precious-gem grinder and seasoned rhinestone producer Laçon, who was himself honored with a gold medal.

At the exhibitions that followed in 1823, 1835, and 1844, Parisian manufacturers of rhinestone and imitation jewelry were always represented. In 1839, at an exhibition of precious metals in London, Bon, a Parisian manufacturer of imitations, created great excitement with his machine-ground rhinestones. At this time, however, he had not yet managed to introduce his grinding machine to a very wide market. This remained for the factories of Swarovsky and Dalloz, and for a time when fashion demanded greater quantities.

Mid-century industrial exhibitions expanded into the international arena. The ambitious Prince Albert instituted the first world exhibition in London in 1851, which was attended by over six million people. In addition to the latest innovations in jewelry materials and their imitations (jet, hair, vulcanized rubber, aluminum, Venetian glass beads, artificial pearls, and so forth), the rhinestone had a strong presence at this great fair, because mass producers were now becoming dominant, often superseding — at least in the case of imitation jewelry — independent workshop and atelier owners. At the Paris exhibition of 1855 thirteen French exhibitors of rhinestone jewelry were present. The German jewelry industry followed suit, and in 1862 at the International Exhibition in London there were twenty-one firms from Pforzheim alone. In 1900 firms from Schwäbisch Gmünd were also represented in Paris.

The concept of the rhinestone as a historical phenomenon first arose at the Exposition Rétrospective de l'Union Centrale des Beaux Arts Appliqués à l'Industrie, which took place in Paris in 1880. Among the items on display were original pieces by Georges Frédéric Stras, and the exhibition gave a clear impression of both the pioneering and the peak periods of this jewelry, which was now at a premium. A new appreciation for old jewelry resulted: it was no longer considered a mere working model or source of inspiration for new designs, but had become a collector's item. It is not without good reason that the Musée des Arts Décoratifs, successor to the Union Centrale des Beaux Arts, owns a significant number of representative rhinestone pieces.

The Twentieth Century: Rhinestones on the International Stage

*B*etween 1910 and 1920 the gradual yet persistent revolution in fashion resulted in the decisive dismissal of the full-length dress from daily wear. This development led to a radical simplification — in comparison with earlier fashions — of ladies' ready-to-wear. Elaborate paddings and inserts to alter the natural fall of material and create complicated draping effects in such styles as the bustle disappeared once and for all. Affected also by the economic crisis and World War I, these definitive changes were rendered irreversible in the twenties, when still more radical forms developed. The "garçonne" style demanded a boyish form, slender shoulders, no emphasis on the bust or waist, and a slim figure with the accent on the vertical line. Aside from their practical use in sports, pants for women gradually became acceptable, particularly in the thirties in the form of the wide-legged divided skirt. And although the leg remained covered, it was still identifiable as such. This was a twentieth-century achievement.

Skirt styles in the twenties allowed the calves, and even the knees, to be visible. As a result, stockings and shoes became a new focal point for fashion accents. Buckles for women's shoes celebrated a comeback, and the rhinestone once again conquered its old domain. In the fifties — as well as today, at the beginning of the nineties — the little glass stone experienced still another heyday, and imitation gems were frequently attached directly to the leather of a shoe. Buckles in the twenties, thirties, and fifties used as a holding device either a crosspiece over a simple square or a double bar (like their eighteenth-century predecessors) or one or more feather clips, an innovation created to beautify the shoe.

As is clear from the example of shoe jewelry, the innovative fashions of the new century did not shy away from ornamentation, even though the styles, with their tendency toward boyishness, were distinctly different from the feminine concepts dominant at the turn of the century. What's more, plain, undraped materials and the lack of ruffles, flounces, extravagant collars, or gathered lace presented unembellished forms that virtually cried out for jewelry. Exposed arms, uncovered throats, and bared ears, made popular by the new sleeveless outfits and short

hairstyles in which the hair was bobbed and swept back in waves, all presented new opportunities for fashion accessories. Long chains — *sautoirs* — which often extended far down the back, necklaces, and *colliers de chien* — chokers made of several strands worn close to the neck and occasionally supplemented with jewelry plaques — were in vogue, as were earrings and ear clips, bracelets for the wrist, and bangles for the upper arm.

But the brooch experienced the greatest revival. In every shape and size imaginable it adorned blouses, jackets, and — the latest thing — the pullover. It turned up on coats, too, and a separate pin for attaching a brooch to a fur coat or collar was constructed with a strong bar-and-clip mechanism. Brooches were also worn as ornamentation on various styles of headdress: caps, toques, berets, turbans, and the oversized hats of the previous century richly endowed with veils, flowers, and ribbons. The pin often served as more than mere decoration; it was used to fasten the veil to the toque or turban cloth as well.

The rhinestone was one of the most popular materials. And it was one of the most important components of evening fashion, which still embraced the full-length dress, although not exclusively. Together with shiny metal sequins, rhinestones, often whole cascades of them, were sewn directly onto such fine materials as silk, lamé, and crepe de chine. In combination with genuine jewelry, rhinestones were thoroughly sufficient to satisfy the requirements of grand evening attire. The close association of genuine and imitation jewelry in the painstakingly distinguished wardrobes of the bourgeoisie during the nineteenth century was shared and revived by a couturiere who was certainly one of the most dazzling and interesting personalities of her profession: Coco Chanel.

Born Gabrielle Chasnel in 1883 in Saumur, France, she opened her first store — a hat shop — in Paris in 1910. Her clientele soon included numerous well-known actresses, but her real breakthrough came with the establishment of her maison de couture in 1915 in Biarritz. It was here that she developed her designs for the simple, short, practical dress, for which she first used jersey — a material reserved until then exclusively for undergarments or sportswear —

and tweed. The little black dress can be traced back to her, as can the street dress, which in decades to come remained a fundamental concept of "Chanel fashion" with only slight variations. She adopted the idea for what was regarded at the time as provocatively short haircuts—the coiffure à la Jeanne d'Arc—from the stage, specifically from her acquaintance with the dancer Caryathis.

As innovative as these changes toward simplicity were, it was never Coco Chanel's objective to revolutionize fashion in the name of social emancipation. She was much too thoroughly integrated into the high society of her time, for which she ultimately worked and in whose circles she traveled. For her, the simple dress demanded luxurious jewelry, so it was not only the exposure of the foot and leg in her fashion designs that shocked traditionalists, but also her juxtaposition of plain day clothes with grand evening jewelry. The "fake" gleam of the rhinestone, faux pearl, and metal struck her as being just right to subvert conventional jewelers' wares. *Bijoux de couture*—costume jewelry—continued to pave the way. In this, too, Chanel was inspired by the stage with its variety shows, revues, and jazz performances, notably Josephine Baker's first famous appearance with the Black Birds dance troupe in 1925.

In Etienne de Beaumont and Duc Fulco di Verdura, Coco Chanel found her most important jewelry designers. Style itself became of greater importance and to some degree even came to overshadow the issue of craft. This was the philosophy of the 1925 Exposition International des Arts Décoratifs in Paris, which turned away from the floral designs of Art Nouveau to endorse a cleaner, more geometric line, creating new possibilities of form and an original, independent design idea for the twentieth century. The cool and austere Art Deco concept was well served by the colorless, transparent stone set in silver; the rhinestone seemed virtually predestined for it.

A multiplicity of sparkling design forms emerged, including all manner of exotica: Africa, primitive tribes, and the Near and Far East were represented, as were ancient Byzantium and Egypt. But unlike the nineteenth century, with its tendency to historicize, the early twentieth century—which to a large extent showed interest in the same areas of art and ethnic tradition—created fashions that did not pretend to imitate the models perfectly, at least as far as clothing was concerned. Exotic models were treated primarily as sources of inspiration for the creation of unique fashion jewelry meant to elicit a strong reaction.

"Fake" materials no longer needed to attempt to conceal themselves but were allowed to display their own intrinsic value.

Synthetic materials benefited most from these changes. In the past there had been increasing experimentation with natural processed products (vulcanized rubber, celluloid, Galalith, and so on), but in 1907 the first fully synthetic material appeared on the market: Bakelite, the invention of the Belgian Leo Hendrik Baekeland. Shortly thereafter came Plexiglas and acrylic, and it is inconceivable today that costume jewelry could have been produced without such synthetics.

Synthetic materials, used in connection with paste and rhinestones, legitimized another fashion designer who was to challenge Coco Chanel's claim to leadership in haute couture in the thirties, and whom Chanel would refer to as *cette modiste* or *l'Italienne*, never by name: Elsa Schiaparelli. Born in 1890 in Rome, Schiaparelli shocked all of Paris not only with her shawls of cellophane and oilcloth, but with numerous other accessories as well, which she considered inseparable from clothing fashion. She designed costume jewelry that consisted primarily of buttons and dainty pins and could be worn anywhere. In 1938 Schiaparelli achieved acclaim for her "circus collection": naive bagatelles such as galloping horses, ostriches, clowns, trapeze artists, and dancers. This was followed by other "theme" collections, including roller skates, bagpipes, leaves, flowers, insects, and little hearts. The circus—a central theme of her work—presented Schiaparelli with a virtually endless source of fantasy and dream motifs. Her ideas helped both clothing and jewelry fashion to establish a strong figural style, and Schiaparelli is frequently credited with having created modern *bijoux de fantaisie*. Of no small influence on her creations were the surrealists Salvador Dalí and Jean Cocteau.

Schiaparelli embroidered lavish pictures onto materials using rhinestones and sequins. Her chromatic effects made with pink, violet, and blue, as well as her colored glass and plastic jewelry, were distinctive. Designers such as Jean Clérmont, Christian Bérard, and, most significantly, Jean Schlumberger worked for her.

The older generation of couturiers had to yield to the advance of costume jewelry and accessories so as not to lose ground entirely. Thus, Paul Poiret, the avant-garde designer responsible for the corsetless dress and divided skirt in the 1910s, permitted glass and ungenuine materials to be used in unique designs, as did his younger colleagues Lucien Lelang and Jean Patou, who were still working as designers into the fifties and sixties.

The effect of costume jewelry had to be even more striking after the grande dame of *bijoux de couture*, Coco Chanel, came out in 1932 with a lavish new collection made exclusively with diamonds—and in countless numbers at that. The collection proved that fashion employing genuine stones could live up to the high standards of costume jewelry design. Something that was to repeat itself in the late eighties had happened: the art of the jeweler and goldsmith became focused on jewelry made of simple and cheap materials once regarded as substitutes for genuine materials, rather than the other way around. This phenomenon, which is recurring now at the close of the twentieth century, is well rooted in tradition.

World War II and the years of deprivation that followed caused a long hiatus in Europe's developing fashion industry, above all in the production of such luxury items as jewelry. It is little wonder that after the years of need and limitation were over everything that had been missed was quickly made up for: an abundance of material and new clothing designs emerged that were not born of a poverty of goods. Ladies' fashions again took a strongly feminine direction, with fitted tops and full, petticoated skirts or the slim-cut "pencil line." Although Christian Dior called his calf-length, full-skirt designs the New Look, the fashion world was not yet ready for any real breakthroughs. Attempts to establish new ideas were marked by a caution that ultimately led to a certain narrow-mindedness, and extreme concepts were regarded with skepticism. The preference for the aesthetically "pretty," that is, for uncomplicated and harmonizing forms, brought a renewed realism to jewelry design: the figural style—which had been introduced in the forties—reached its peak. Cheap materials commonly replaced genuine ones and rhinestones replaced diamonds, though without the tension between genuine jewelry and costume jewelry that had reigned in the twenties and thirties. The joy of being able to indulge oneself with attractive ornaments seemed to be all that mattered. And sparkling stones began to appear in every conceivable place, including eyeglass frames, lipstick cases, and cigarette holders.

It is no accident that during the fifties and even more so since the sixties a new branch of jewelry design split off from the traditional goldsmith's art: the avant-garde, which was consciously seeking to free itself from previous and newly revived conventions. Regarding itself as a true art, this new movement rejected mass production and formed a new, third direction in jewelry design. For the avant-garde, the past was just as valuable a resource as the many variations of both natural and artificial materials.

But the rhinestone remained, as before, the domain of costume jewelry, which, with the renewed and increasing design consciousness of the sixties, once again took center stage, most of all in association with the "hippie" fashion of long chains and extravagant earrings. Polystyrene synthetics presented a genuine rival to past imitations, because the technique of injection molding, to which this type of plastic lent itself very well, boosted mass production greatly. This technique, more than any other, made use of the cheap labor of certain countries, such as Taiwan and Korea, which are now the primary producers of mass-produced wares sold internationally at low prices. Plastic poured into facet molds began to appear as substitute rhinestones, turning the paste of the past—once the cheapest variation—into a luxury item, since its production was so much more complicated. Even the settings of such jewelry items are injected or poured, and the plastic stones are simply pressed in.

The rhinestone that again became an obligatory component of haute couture jewelry and accessories in the late eighties is, of course, of the "genuine" variety, produced with care and made into every conceivable form, size, and setting. In the best postmodern manner no single style predominates; on the contrary, every style is permitted, resulting in an eclectic collective image, the only requirement for which is that it all glitter. One of the most favored makers of such high-fashion rhinestone jewelry is Kenneth Jay Lane in New York.

The United States Acquires the Rhinestone: American Rhinestone Factories

At the beginning of this century the rhinestone made its way to the New World, landing on such fertile ground that the history of its production and manufacture, everything known about the hundred-fifty-year-old gem, was cast into obscurity.

In the 1940s in the area of New York and Providence, Rhode Island, alone, there were over nine hundred firms specializing in costume jewelry, rhinestone jewelry in particular. Some of the oldest firms are Coro (actually Cohn & Rosenberger), founded in 1902, and Albert Weiss, who originally worked with Coro and opened his own enterprise in 1942. Some of the most well-known include Eisenberg (founded in 1914; after 1942 known as Eisenberg Ice) and Trifari (actually Trifari, Krussmann & Fischel). Mamie Eisenhower appeared wearing Trifari jewelry at her husband's inauguration ball in 1952 and duped the fashionable conservatives there with her imitations. Eisenberg pieces using Swarovsky-made stones belong to the most sought-after collectors' pieces because of their meticulous prewar sterling silver settings and postwar rhodium-plated settings. A few more names bear mention: Hobé, Bogoff, Vendôme, Napier, Myriam Haskell, Joseff of Hollywood, and Kramer. Craftsmen from France and Italy who emigrated to the United States frequently found employment in these firms.

But America had and indeed still has no predominant fashion center on the order of Paris; still, it is endowed with an institution that can, to a certain degree, be described as an emporium for the latest fashion trends: Hollywood. Among other things, the film industry took over the role that nineteenth-century theater had played, becoming a showplace for new fashion designs. Whereas in the past fashion houses competed for commissions to create costumes for the great stage actresses, today designers vie to dress the leading screen actresses and have their names appear in the film credits. The relative fame of the actress serves as a special signal, a kind of advertising to show what, when, and how things should be worn.

Clothing and jewelry fashion were in the limelight especially during Hollywood's heyday, from the thirties to the fifties, when entire scripts were written around popularly acclaimed actresses. It is no accident that both Chanel and Schiaparelli turned up in Hollywood to design costumes. The great expansion in American costume jewelry firms that occurred at the end of the thirties was certainly due in part to the influence of Hollywood's golden age.

On the screen, imitation jewelry was called upon to create an appearance of luxury. This was especially true of historical films, which required elaborate costumes. Historical styles of jewelry consequently found acceptance with movie audiences and began to appear as fashion accessories available in stores. Whether Greta Garbo or Marlene Dietrich portrayed historical figures, such as Queen Christina or Catherine the Great, or present-day characters, their impressive images encouraged imitation. The major rhinestone manufacturers complied, producing a multitude of motifs and styles that surpassed the pretenses of the French *bijoux de couture* and *bijoux de fantaisie* and were based directly on lavish rococo designs. It seems impossible today to speak of anything that has not already been done in an earlier time and place. The motives behind the production of rhinestone jewelry in America can be read as a condensed version of the entire history of the rhinestone.

Plates

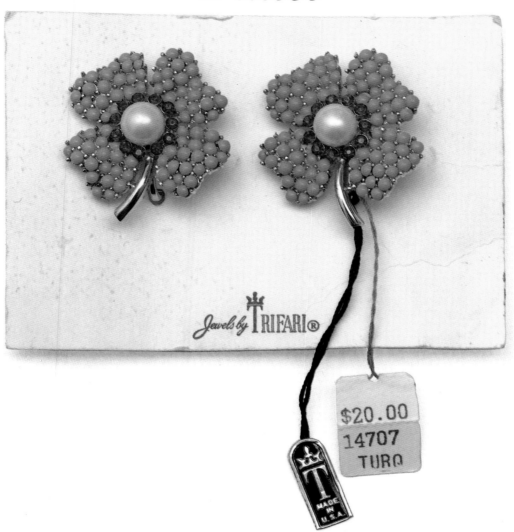

*E*arrings, signed Trifari, in their
original packaging, 1940

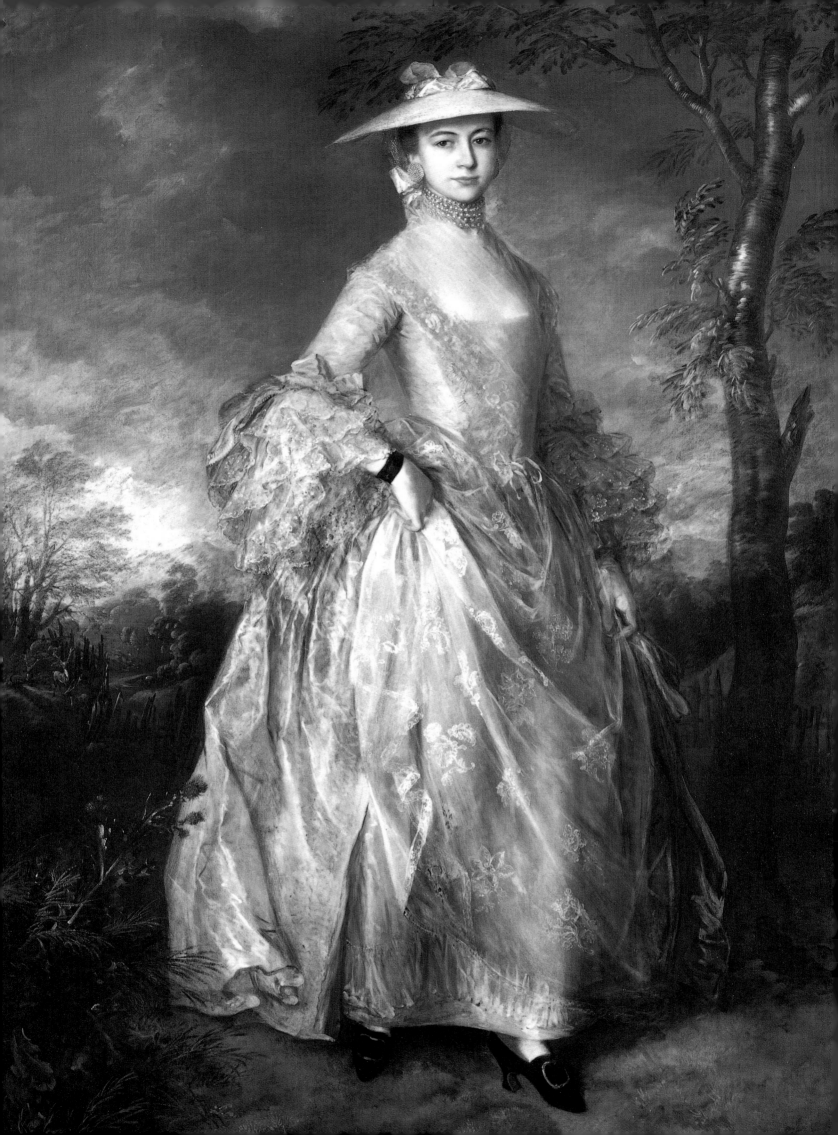

Shoe Buckles

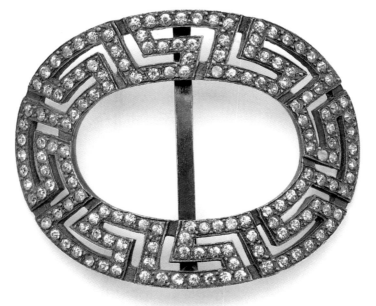

S how your dainty feet, show your shoes!" Noble ladies and gentlemen once proudly decorated their elegant pumps with glittering buckles. Rhinestones gave the shoe a regal air. And today films reel off the history of fashion. Long live Amadeus! A ponytail, a buckle twinkling against black velvet—dangerous liaisons lead to temptation—even if it's all only for the sake of a gleam. Authentic ornamental buckles of the ancien régime are true showpieces of the jeweler's art and coveted rarities to boot.

Shoe buckles in the classical meandering design, rhinestones set in silver, 1770

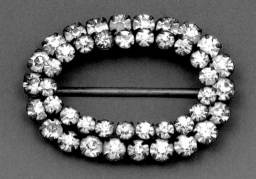

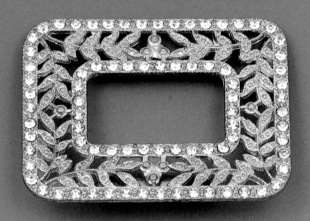

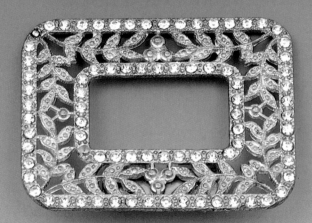

*TOP: shoe buckle with double row of
large round rhinestones, 1780
BOTTOM: pair of matching shoe buckles,
white rhinestones, produced
in Hollywood, 1930*

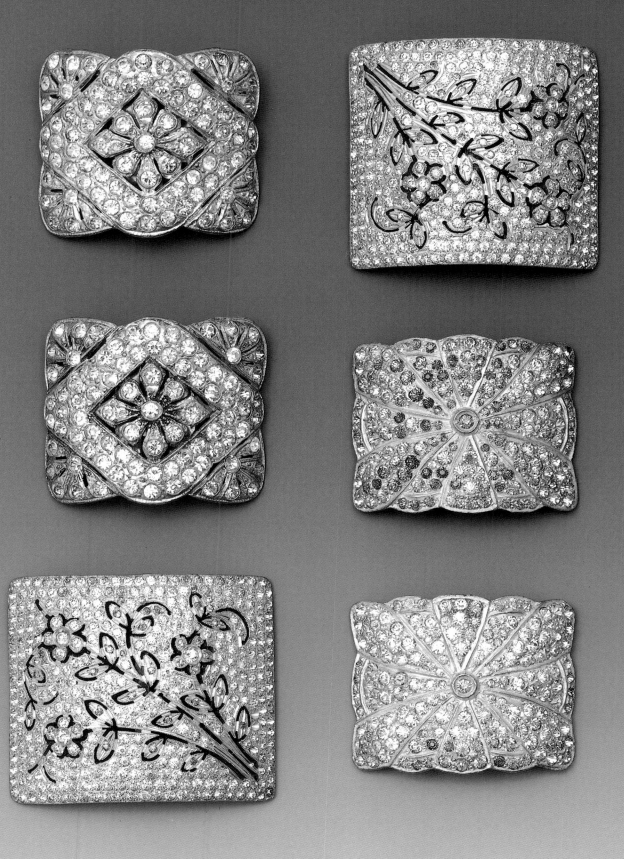

Three pairs of decorative Hollywood shoe buckles, 1930

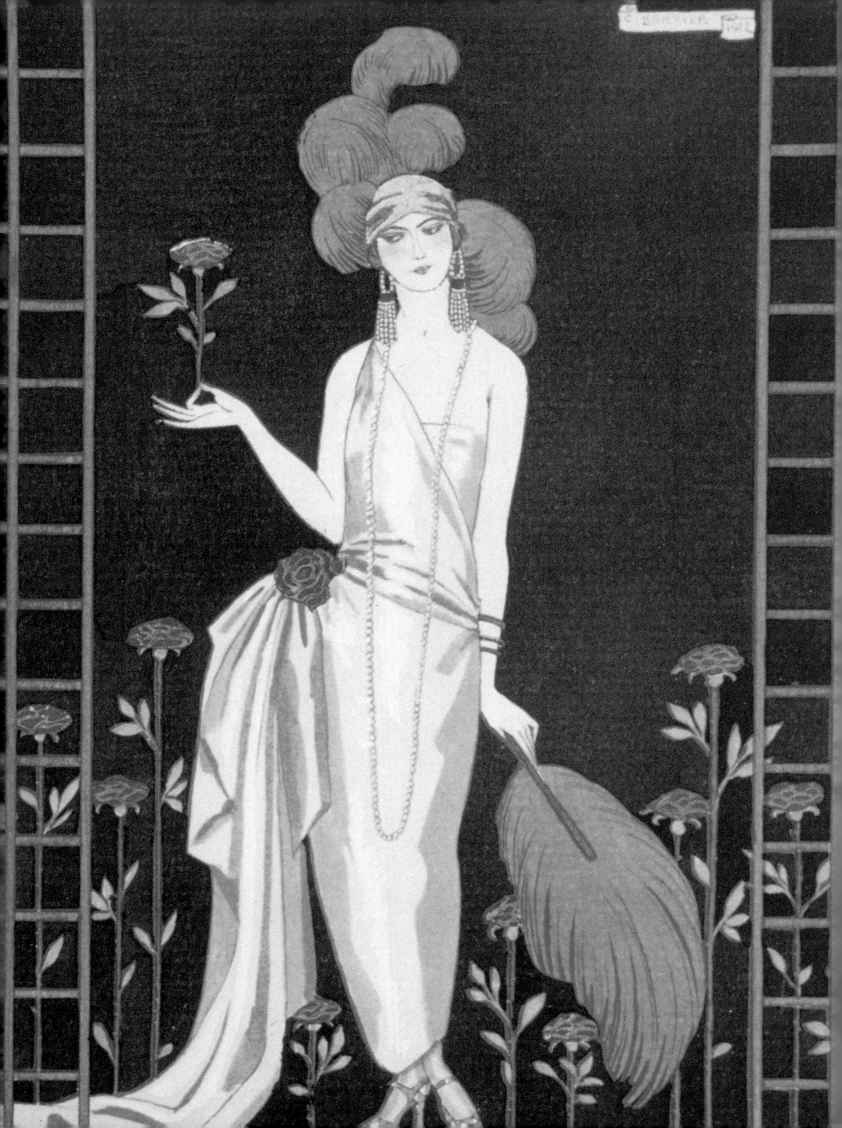

Flowers

*S*parkling calyxes, opulent blossoms, dainty floral clusters—a breath of spring for every season. Flora's dream garden as a coquettish center of attention on the ear and at the throat, favorite jewelry of years gone by, when a woman in veil and gloves was still considered a perfect lady and liberation was yet in its infancy. The playful charm of earrings and brooches, whose sensual combination of cool glass, brilliant colors, and stylized form still enchants. The language of flowers again entices the play of contrasts and is timelessly appealing in its charm and elegance.

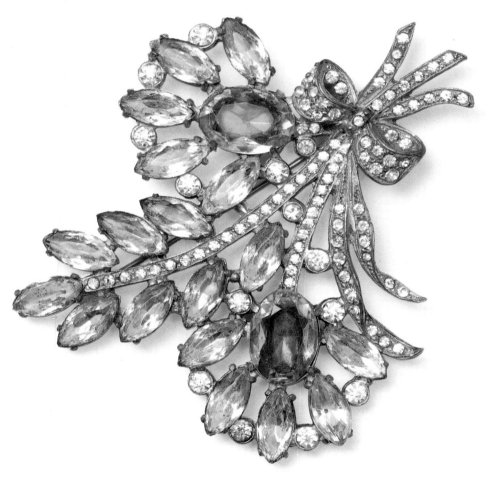

*B*rooch worn diagonally, floral spray gathered with a bow, white and colored rhinestones, 1938

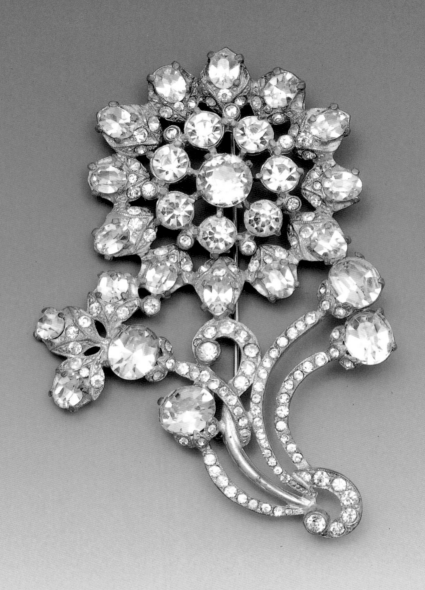

*F*ull-blossomed flower and closed buds,
white rhinestones set in white metal, 1935

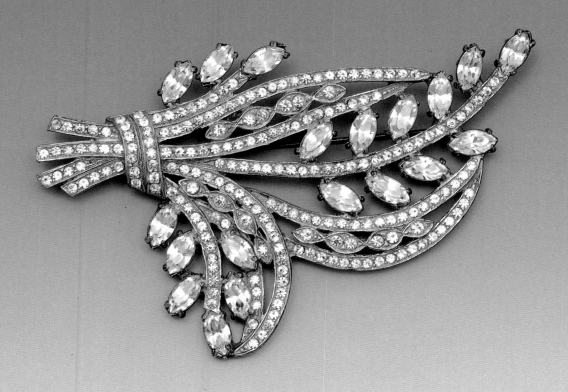

Sheaf of wheat, rhinestones, 1935

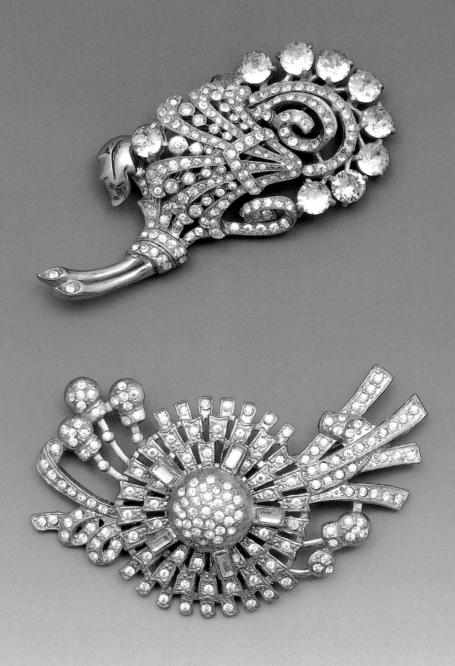

*T*OP: *rhinestone floral spray set in gold-*
and silver-colored metal, 1940
*B*OTTOM: *circular rhinestone flower on*
gold-colored metal, 1935

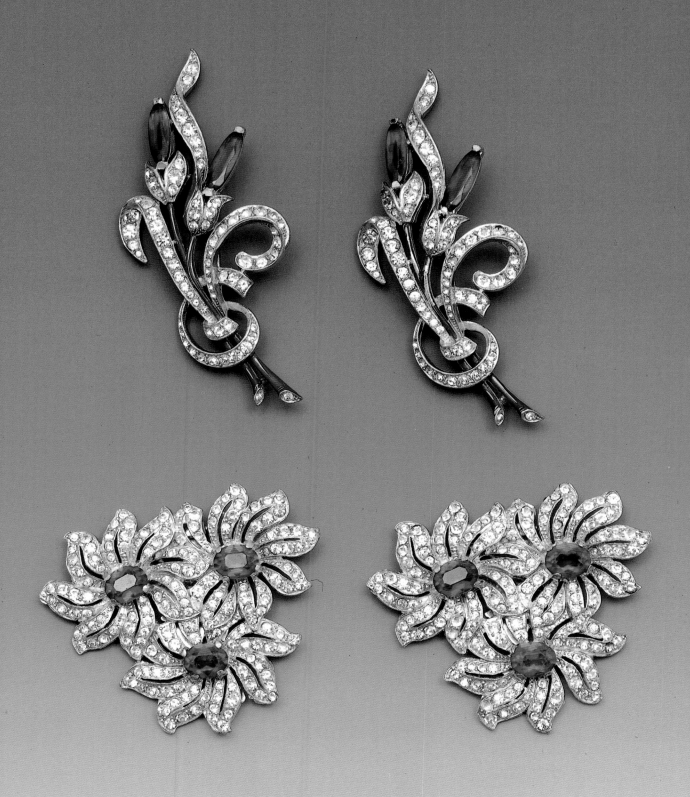

*TOP: pair of unusual brooches, signed
Trifari, 1939
BOTTOM: pair of rhinestone clothing
clips, each of three flowers, 1935*

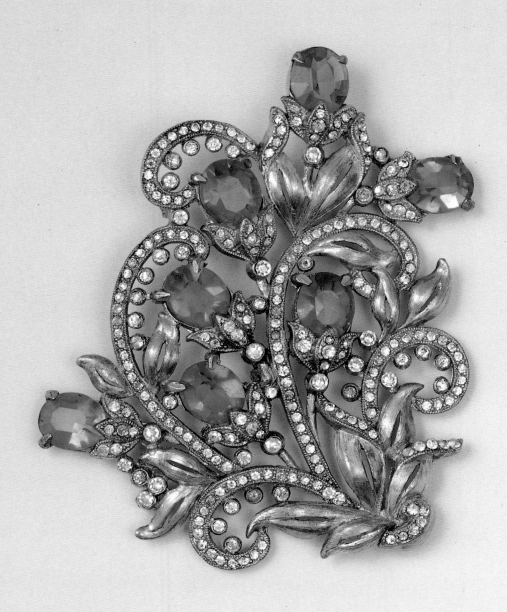

*A*BOVE: *flower petal brooch, white
rhinestones with blue glass, 1935*
OPPOSITE, TOP: *sheaf of wheat,
rhinestones with colored glass, 1940*
BOTTOM: *floral spray brooch, 1940*

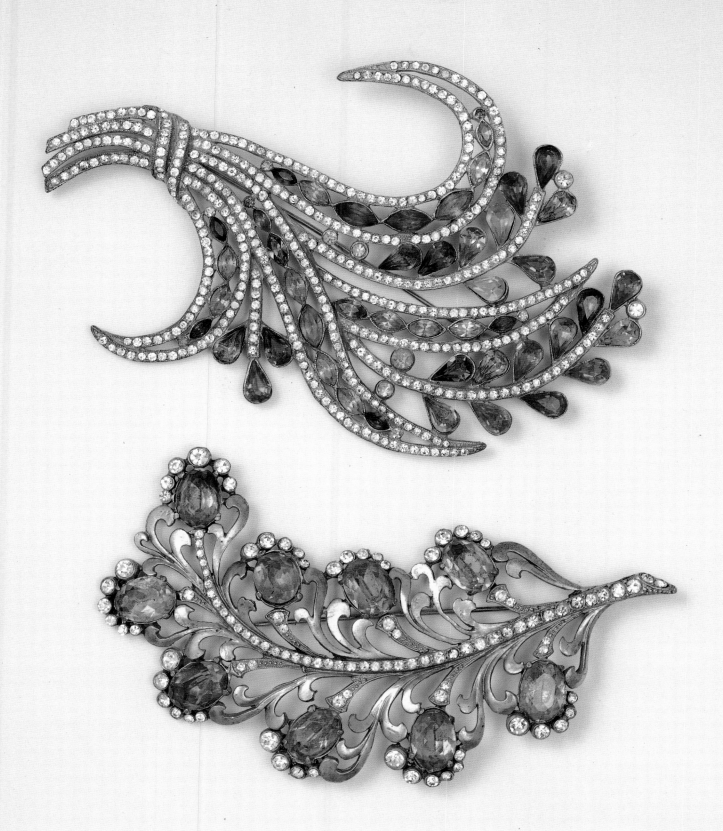

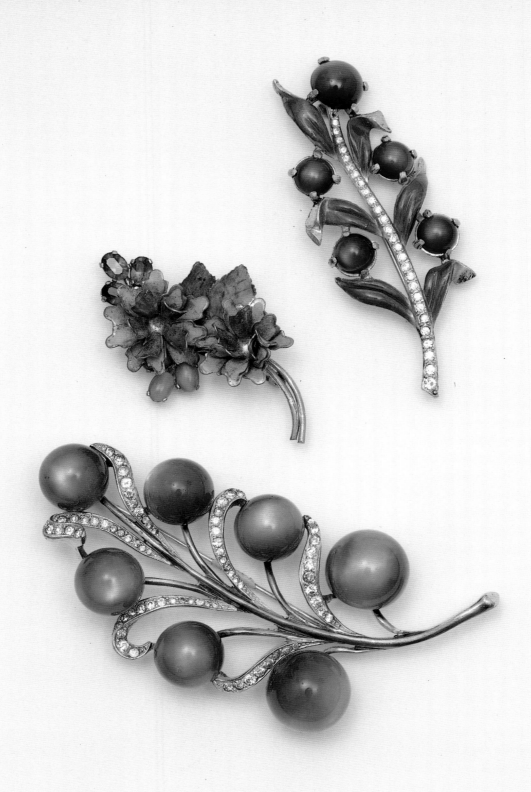

*T*OP: *rhinestone spray with red
stones, 1942*
CENTER: *floral spray, rhinestones and
painted metal, 1930*
BOTTOM: *brooch, rhinestones combined
with moonstonelike glass cabochons, 1942*
OPPOSITE: *"Coro Duettes": pins fastened
to double clips, allowing them to be
separated and worn individually; each
piece signed* Coro Duette, *1940*

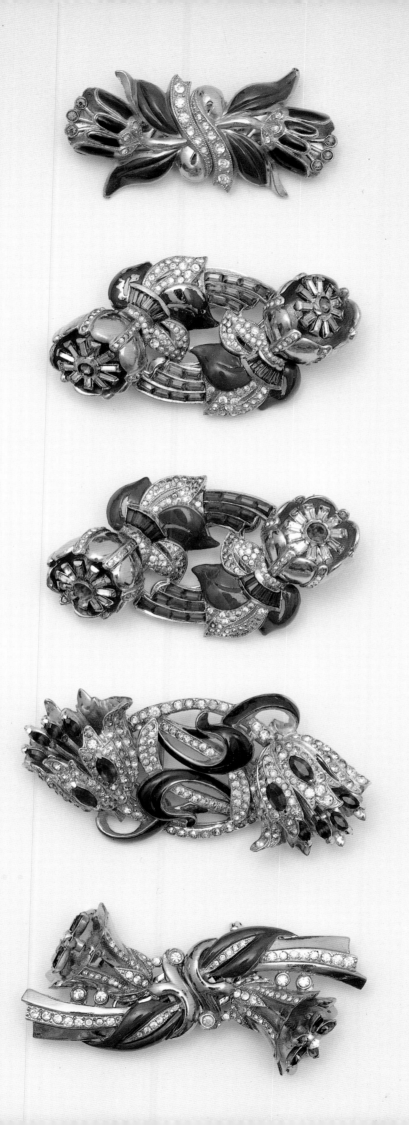

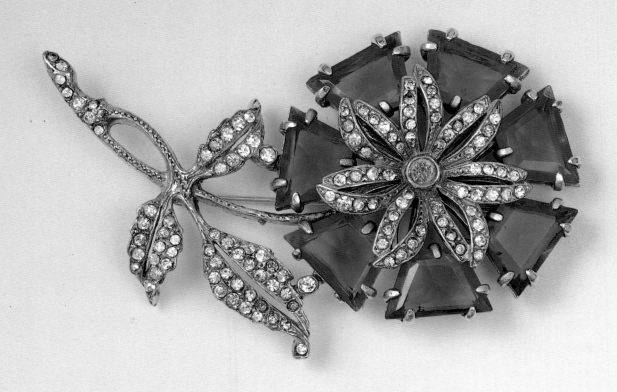

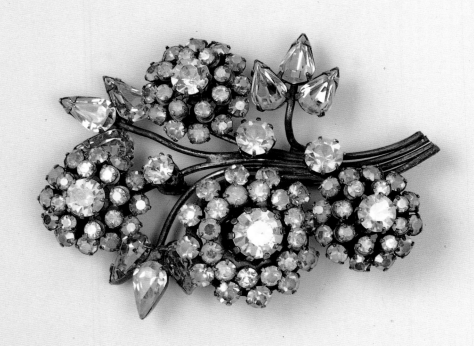

*T*OP: *large flower brooch, rhinestones*
with three-corner-cut blue stones, signed
Reinard, *1935*
*B*OTTOM: *floral spray brooch of*
iridescent rhinestones, signed
Vendôme, *1950*

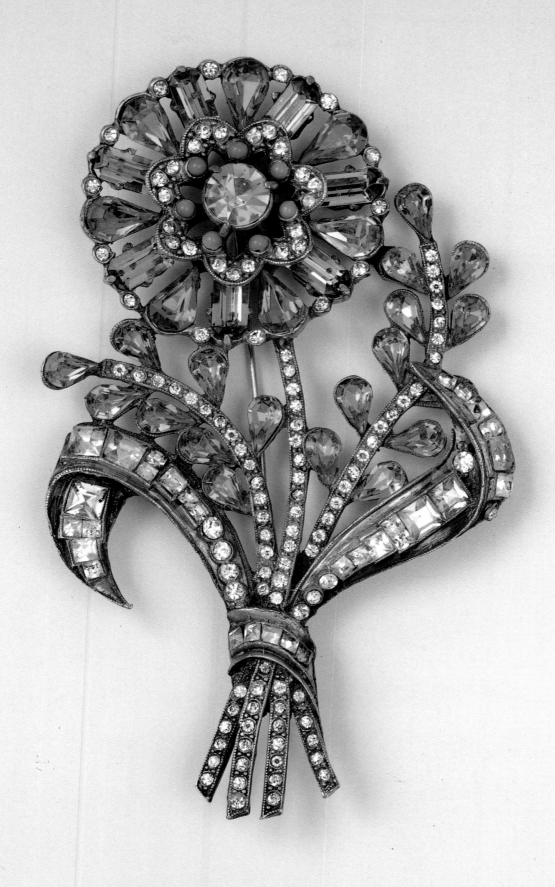

*Extraordinarily large, turquoise-colored
flower with sprays and leaves, signed
Staret, 1940*

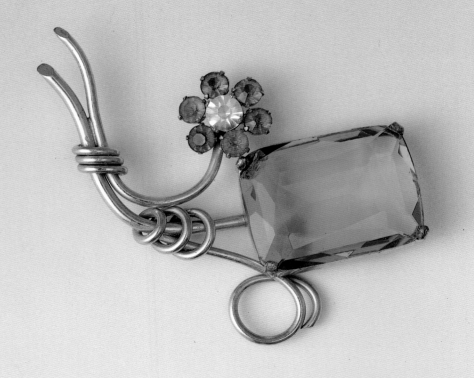

*A*BOVE: *pin, rhinestones and unusually
large light green stone, signed*
Les Glass, *1950*
*O*PPOSITE: *various rhinestone floral
spray pins, 1950–55*
*T*OP, LEFT: *an exceptionally striking
nosegay pin, signed* Coro, *1950*

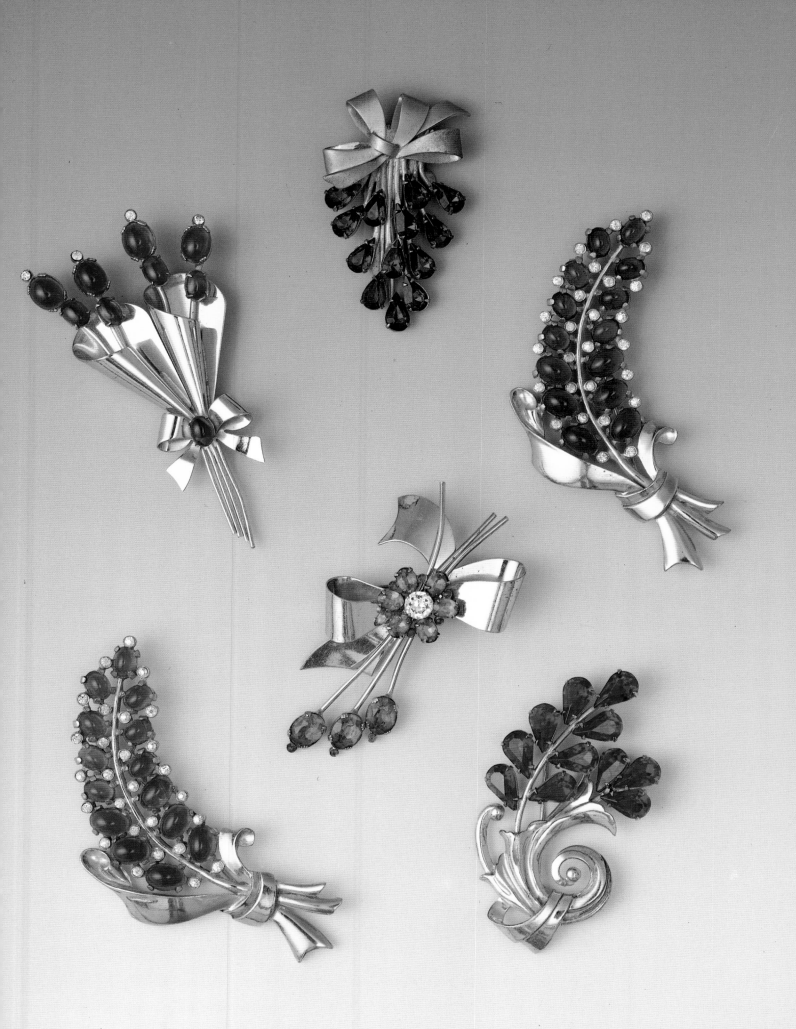

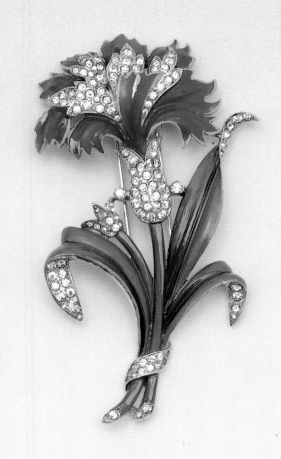

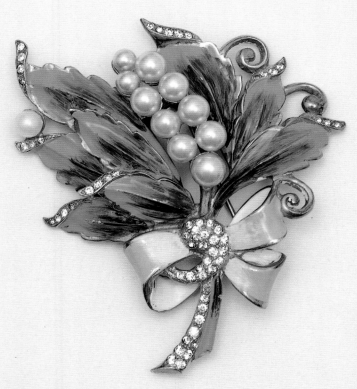

*T*OP: *pin, signed* Trifari, *1940*
BOTTOM: *rhinestone clip, signed* Reja, *1940*
OPPOSITE, TOP: *heavy, downward-*
hanging flower pin, 1940
CENTER: *pin with pearled lilies, 1935*
BOTTOM: *lily-of-the-valley pin, signed* Coro, *1940*

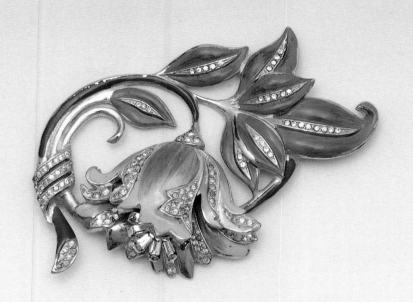

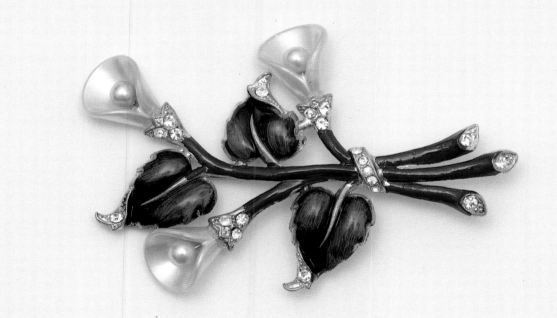

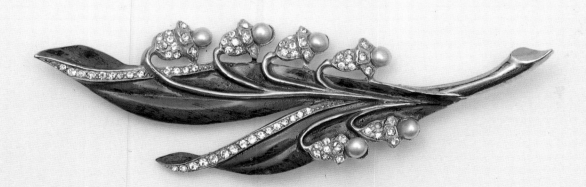

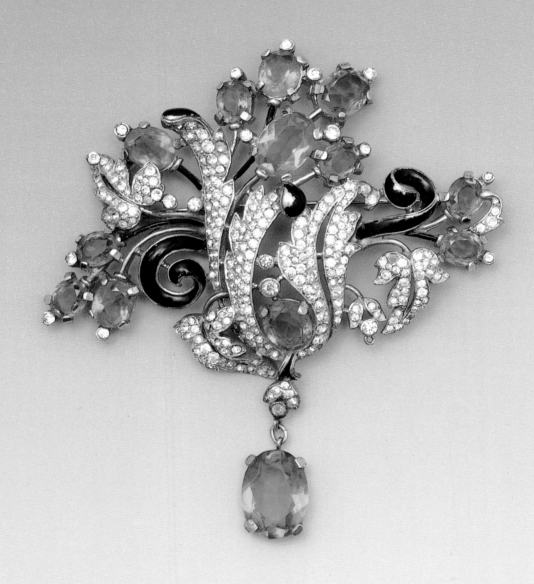

*Extraordinary rhinestone brooch in the
form of a sumptuous bouquet with
hanging pendant, 1935*

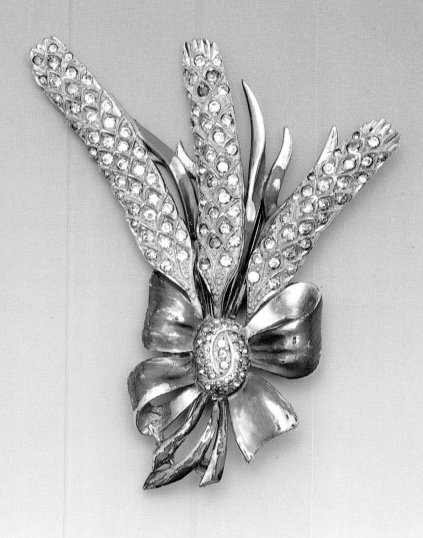

*Brooch in the form of corncobs gathered
with a bow, 1940*

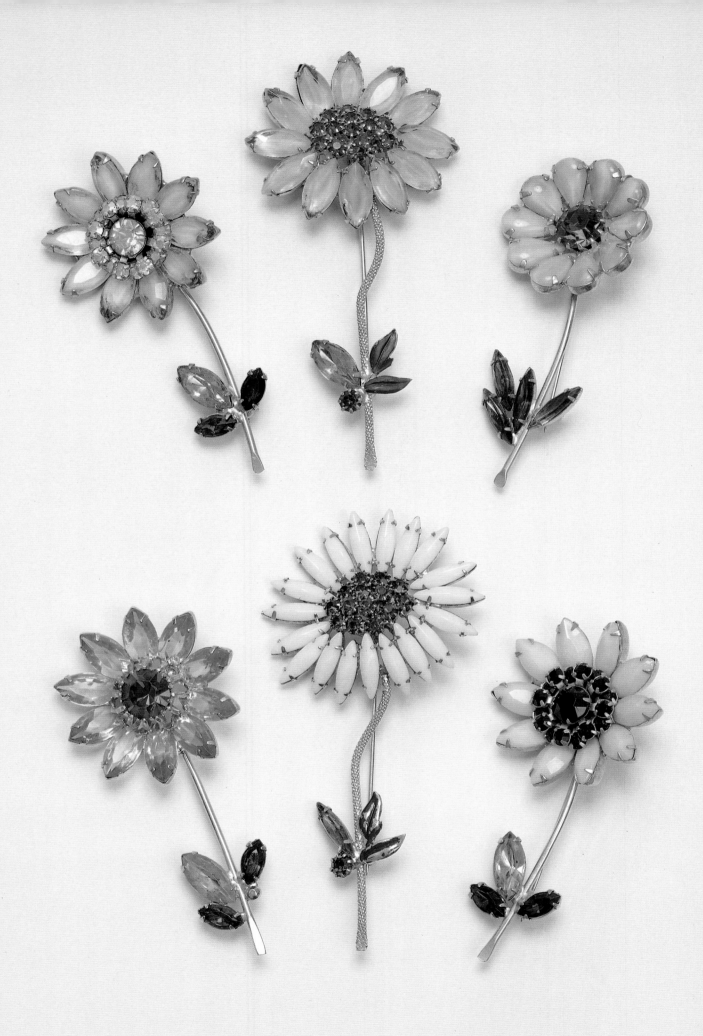

Pins in various classical flower shapes,
all signed Weiss

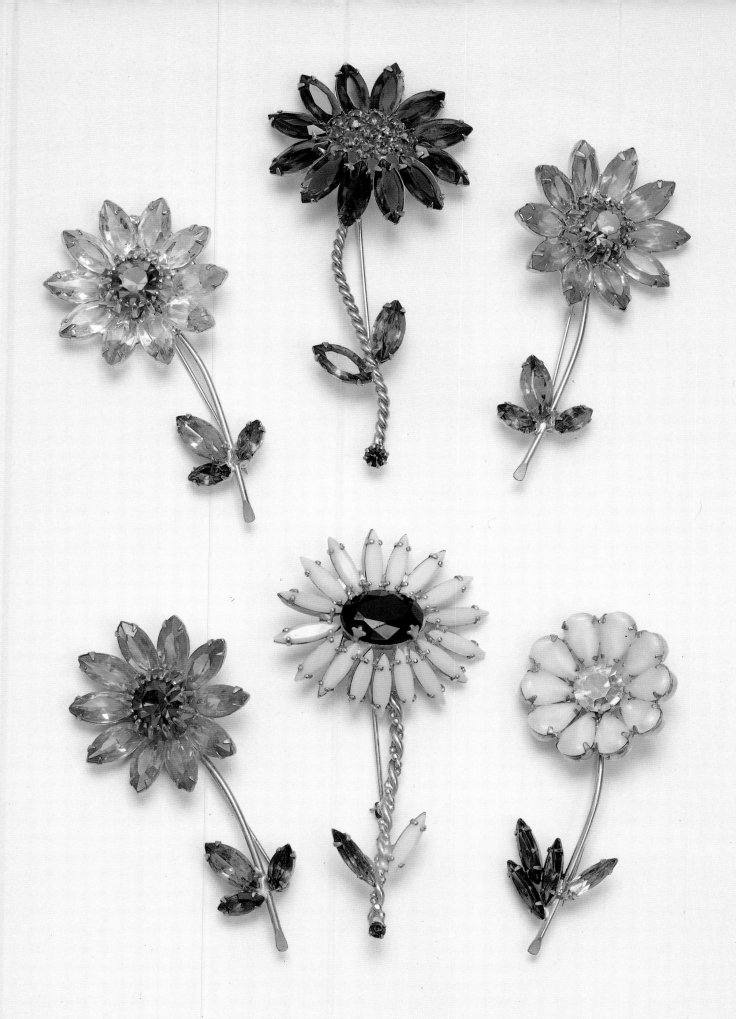

*A harvest of rhinestone flower pins,
with stems and petals partially of metal
or colored glass, all 1950*

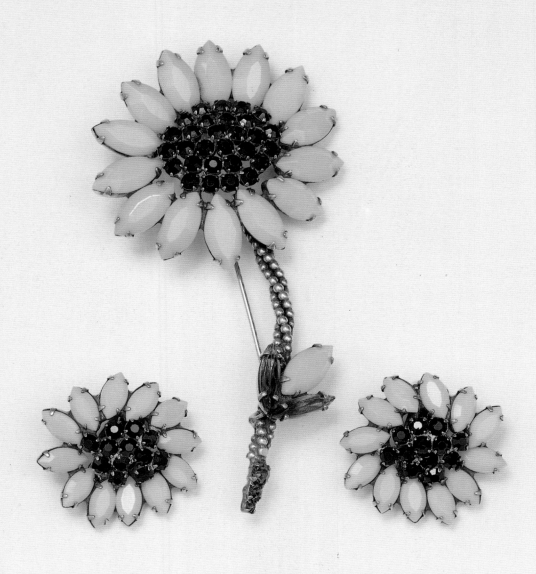

*Two sets of blossom pins with matching
earrings by Weiss*

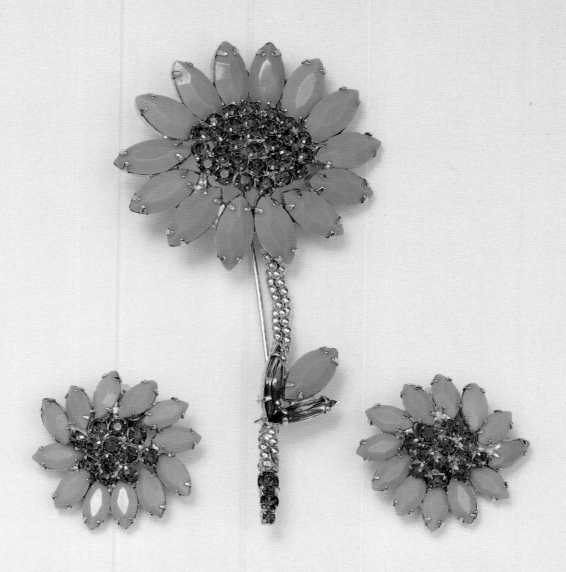

*The flower centers and stem ends are of
rhinestones, the petals of colored glass;
both sets 1950*

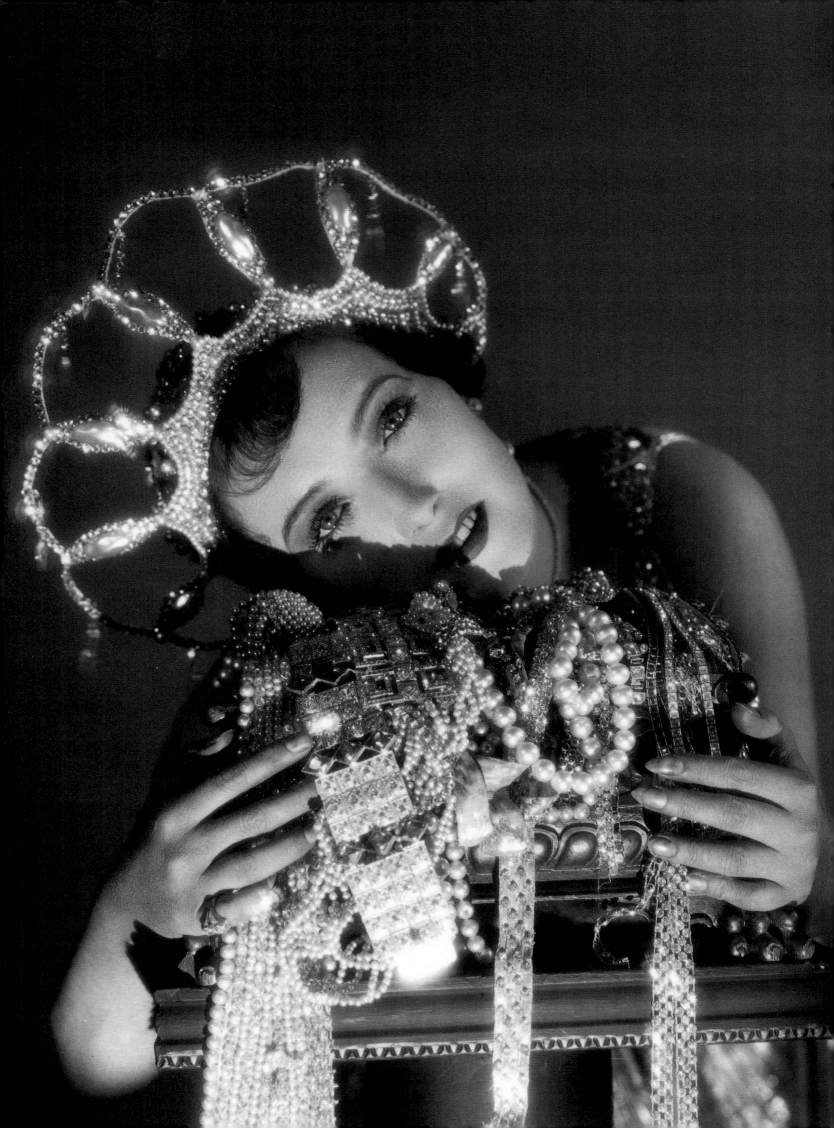

Curiosities

*T*here is a wonderful light-hearted side to the rhinestone. It invites playfulness, experimentation with form and fantasy. It can be made into ephemeral jewelry, permitting all kinds of quirkiness: kitsch and trinkets, exotica, curiosities, and amusements. With a twinkle in their eye designers present their creations: wedding carriages, circus elephants, elegant ladies, Mississippi steamboats. One can uncover a hint of the spirit of the times in such a piece—or experience a piece of history just by wearing it.

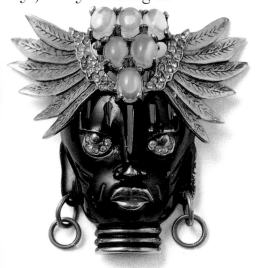

So-called Blackamoor, rhinestones on stained sterling silver, signed Reja, *1938*

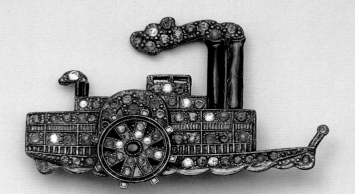 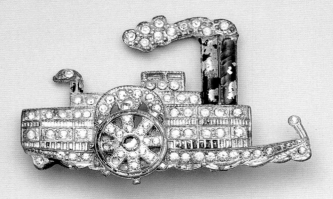

Two steamboats with movable wheels,
rhinestones on metal, 1935

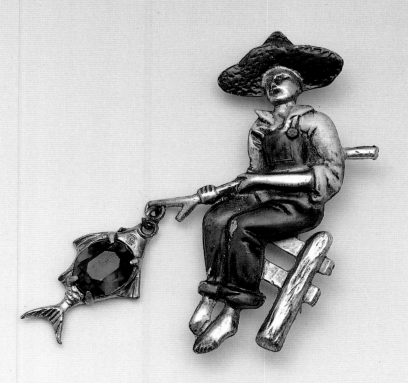

Huckleberry Finn with fishing pole,
pin, rhinestone and colored glass, 1930

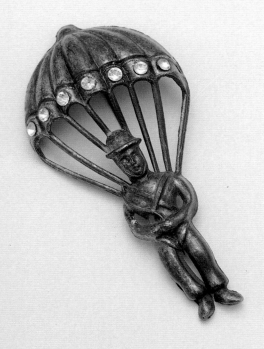

*A*BOVE: *landing parachutist, pin, 1930*
*O*PPOSITE: *coach and covered wagon with
moving wheels, rhinestones on white
metal, both 1930*

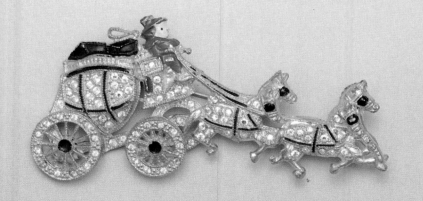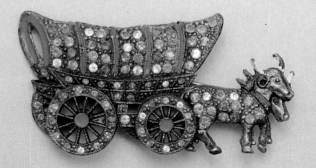

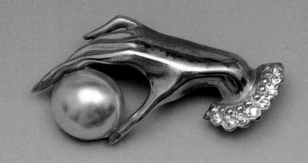

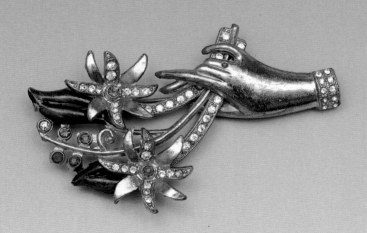

*Top: hand with pearl and rhinestone
cuff, pin, 1953
Bottom: hand with floral spray, metal
set with rhinestones, 1940*

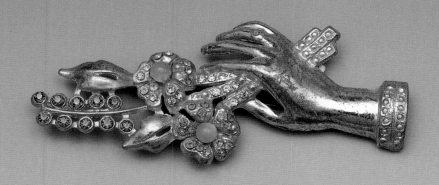

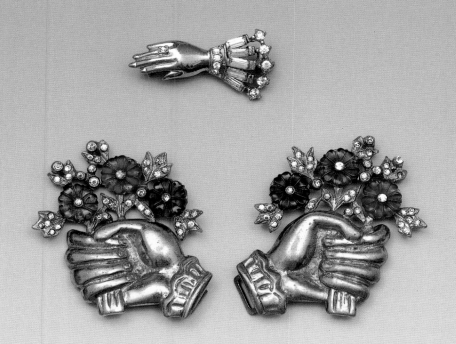

*T*OP: *hand with rhinestone bouquet,*
pin, 1935
*C*ENTER: *hand with rhinestone ring and*
rhinestone cuff, 1935
*B*OTTOM: *belt buckle with rhinestone*
bouquets, 1900

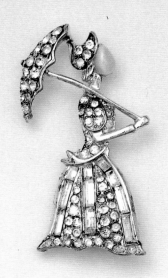

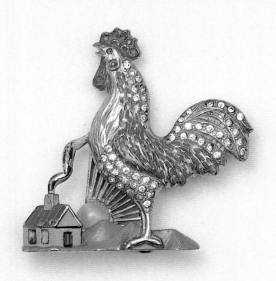

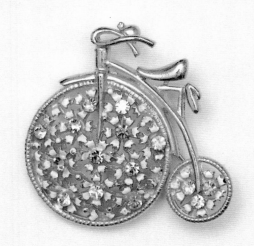

*T*OP: *rhinestone lady with parasol, 1940*
CENTER: *rhinestone rooster in*
foreground of house with smoking
chimney, pin, 1940
BOTTOM: *bicycle with colored*
rhinestones, 1955

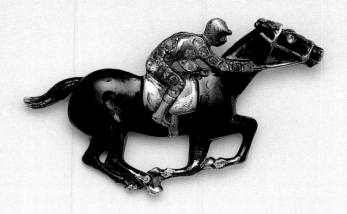

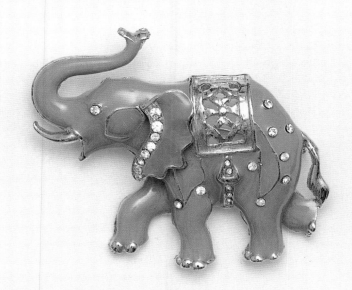

*T*op: *galloping horse with jockey,
pin, 1935*
*B*ottom: *marching elephant, pin,
rhinestones on plastic, 1935*

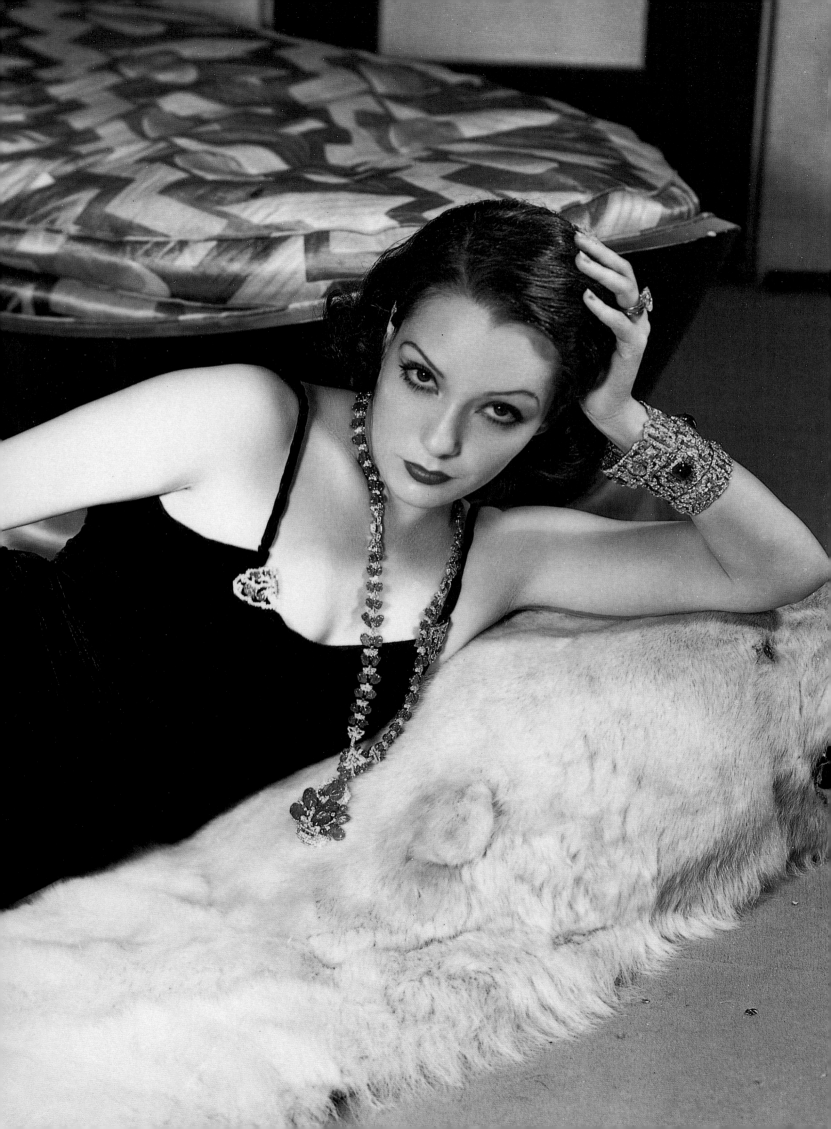

Leaves

*M*emories of summer sunlight on long promenades, of winding paths canopied with rustling leaves, of the joy of the first buds of spring: euphemism and suggestion alike, brought

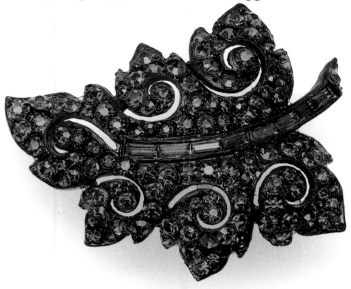

together in myth and fairy tale, are transformed into pieces of jewelry. Fragile images—fixed forever. White and deep green rhinestones, as diversely formed as their natural counterparts. As though "gone with the wind," they drift down and land in the hair, on the shoulder. Striking accessories, individually or gathered in bunches, lavishly decorated or as gleaming metallic frames for a sparkling stone. Old faithfuls are interpreted in surprising new ways, while the charm of the symbol endures.

*R*hinestone leaf, green stones on black
lacquered metal, 1940

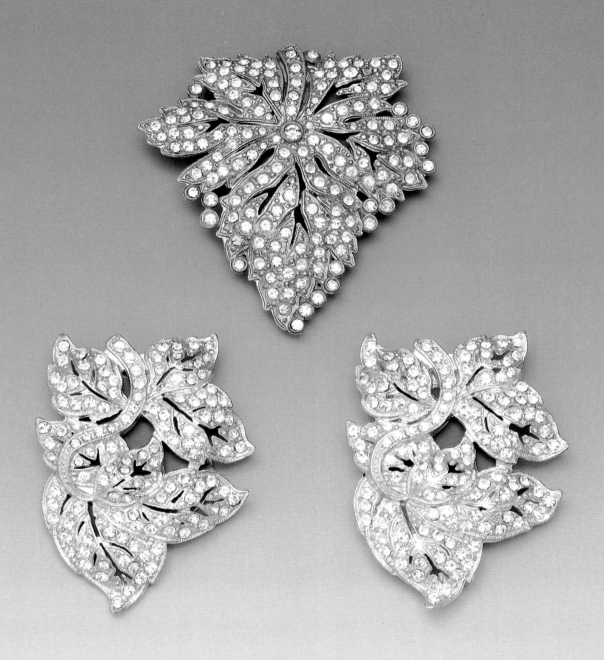

*T*OP: *leaf clothing clip, white*
rhinestones, 1935
*B*OTTOM: *pair of leaf clothing clips,*
white rhinestones, 1935

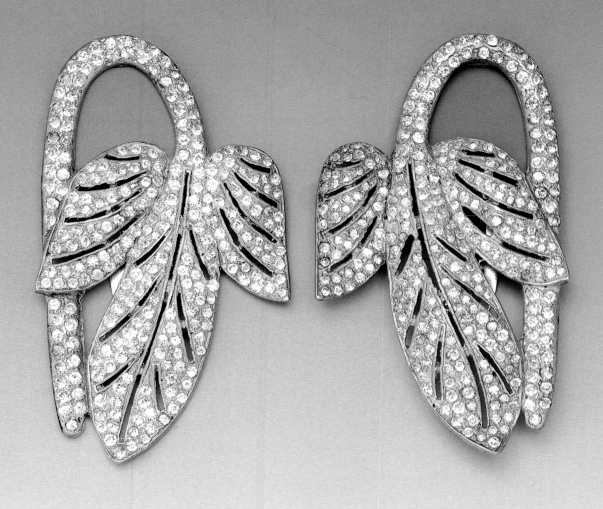

*P*air of large leaf clothing clips, white
rhinestones, 1935

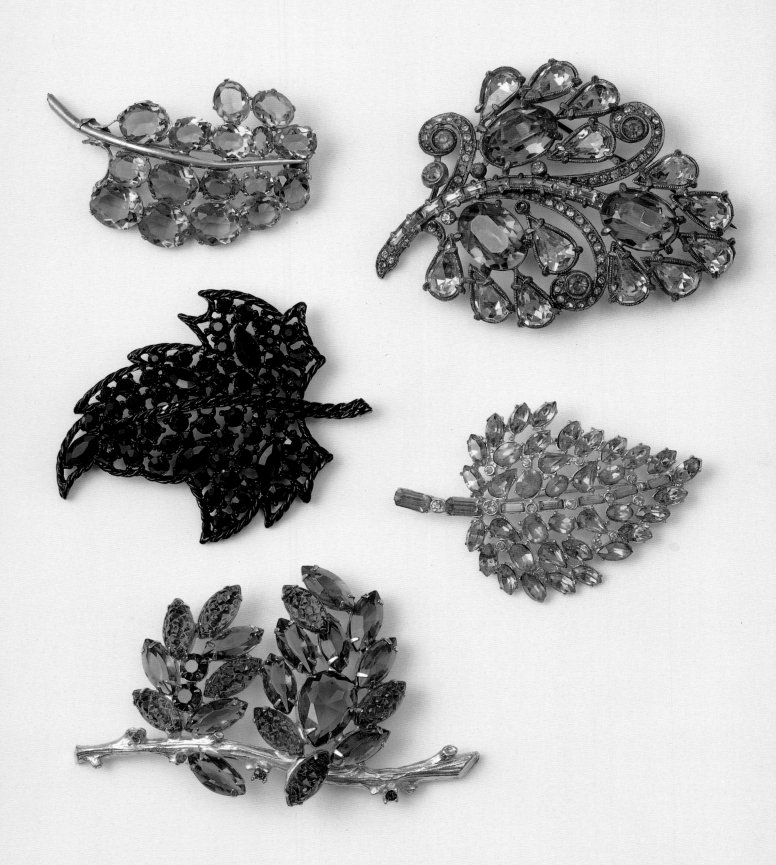

Various rhinestone leaf pins, 1930–40

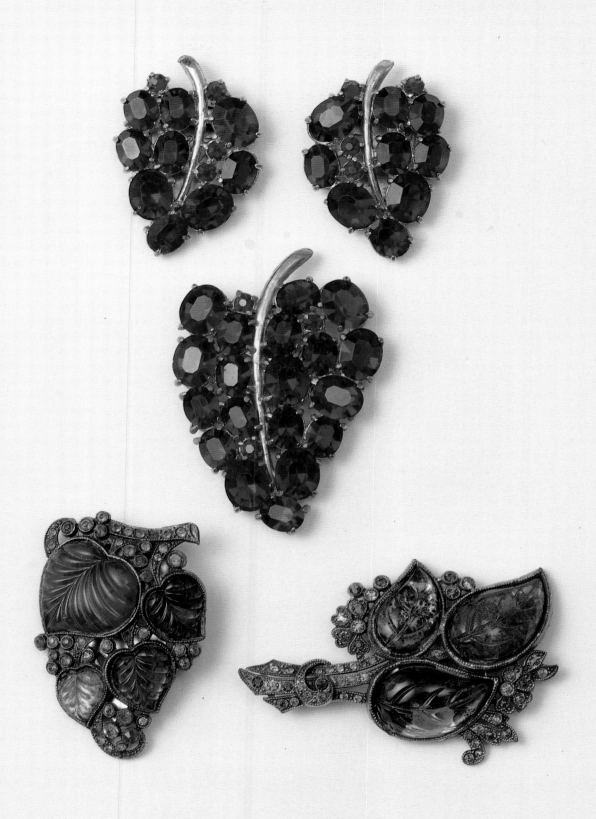

Clothing clips, rhinestones on brass, 1938

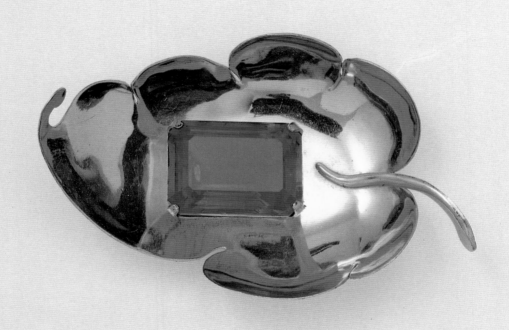

*Large leaf with single stone set in
gold-colored silver, signed Coro, 1940*

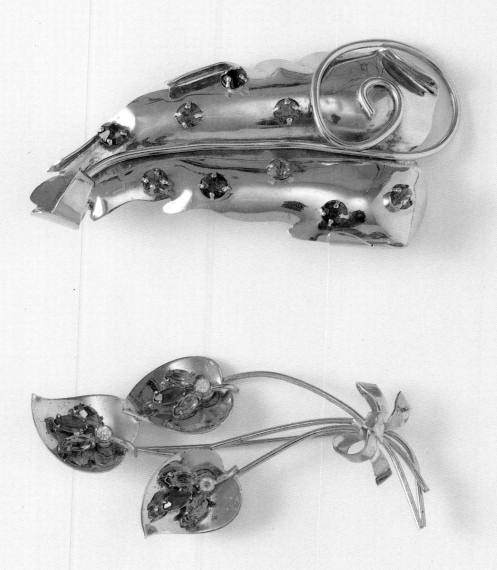

TOP: rhinestone leaf, gold-colored
sterling silver, 1938
BOTTOM: small leaves gathered in a
bouquet, rhinestones on gold-colored
sterling silver, signed Coro, 1940

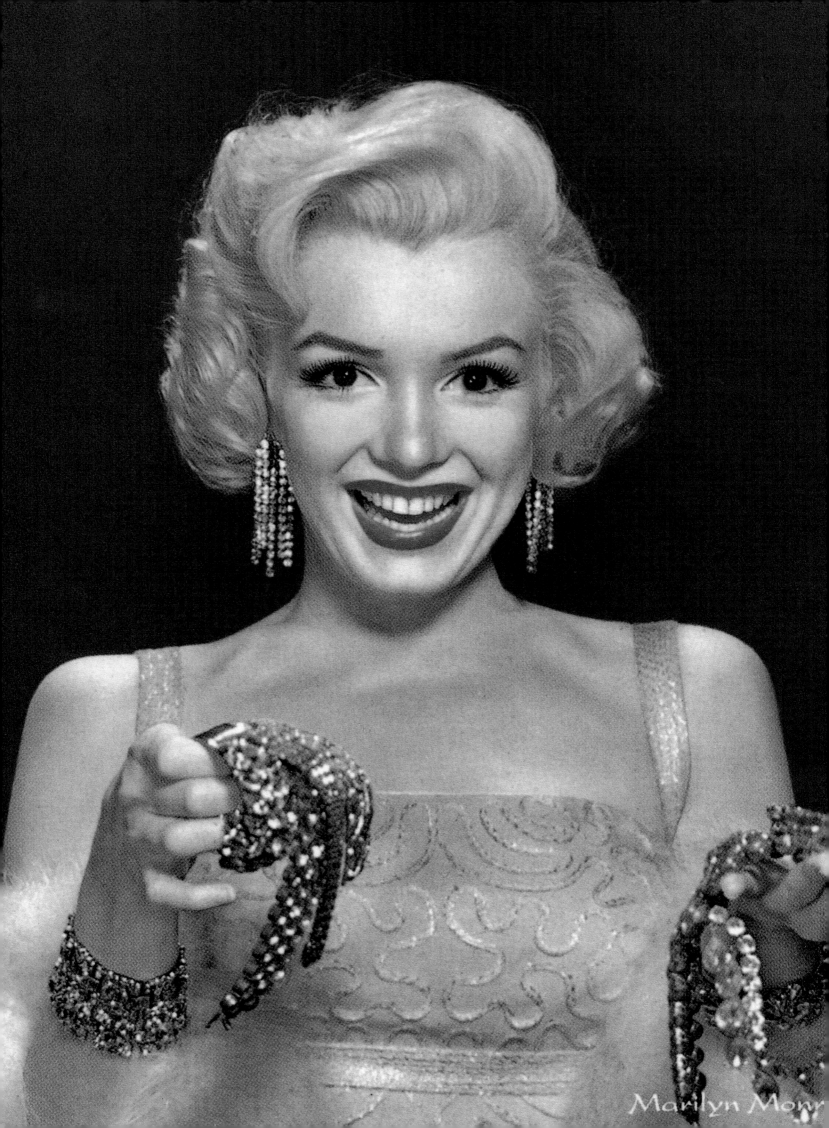

Marilyn Monr

Necklaces and Bracelets

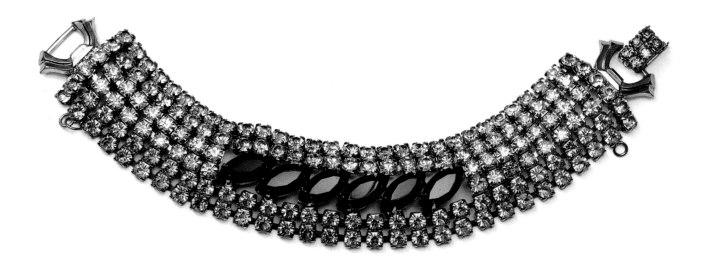

Some like it hot . . . Two, three bracelets on each wrist, necklaces, earrings. In jewelry sets two plus two equals more than four. The play of complementary pieces creates fireworks. Marilyn was successful with her artful bait. But even solo the luxurious jewels lose not a bit of their effect: baroque baubles and bangles on long, black gloves, delicate chains against bare skin. The art lies in subtle variations — the philosophy of the rhinestone makes it possible.

Bracelet, signed Weiss; at its center black marquise stones, 1940

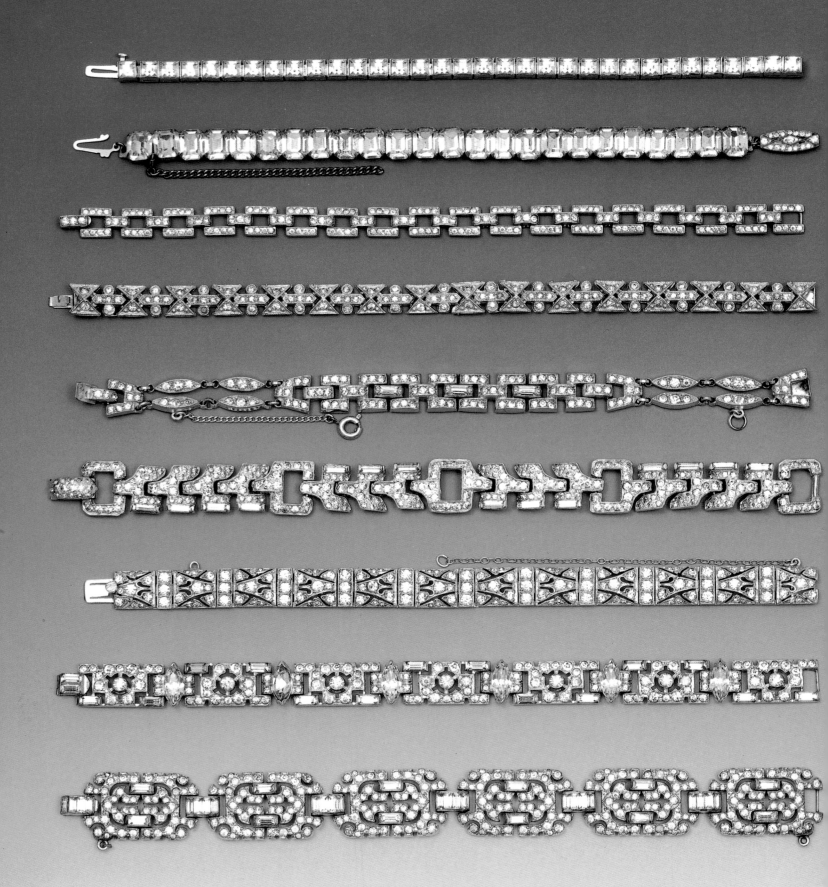

White rhinestone bracelets
TOP: *rhinestones set in sterling silver;
signed* Dowsons, *1940*
SECOND FROM TOP: *signed* Weiss, *1940*
THIRD FROM TOP: *rhinestones set in
sterling silver, signed* Trifari, *1940*
BOTTOM: *last two bracelets signed* TKF,
both 1935

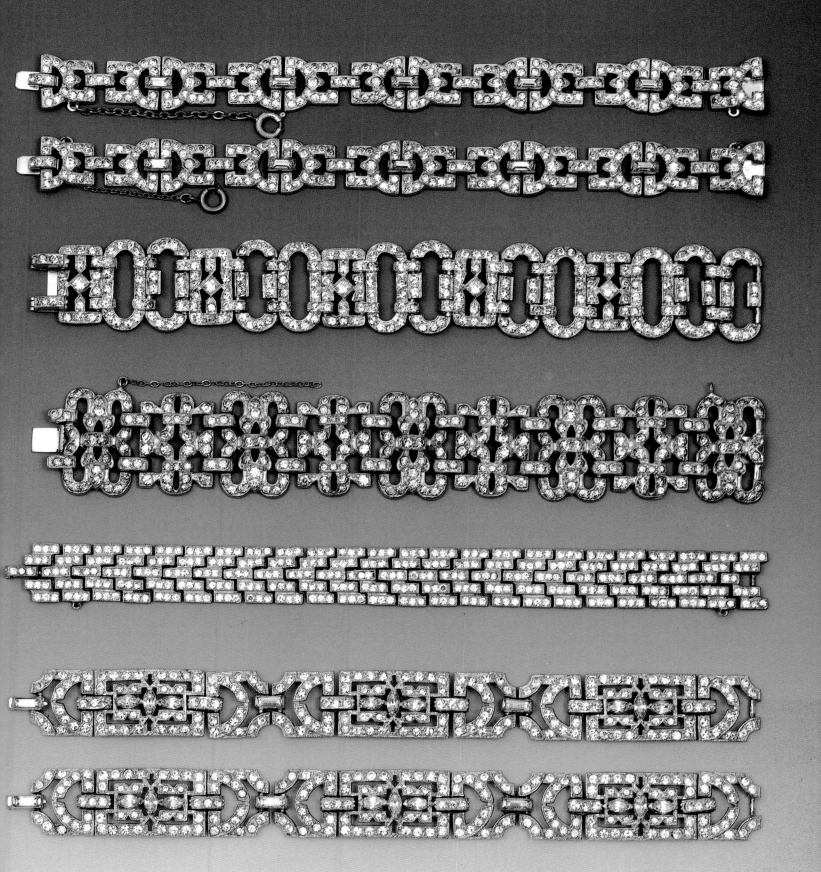

*White rhinestone bracelets, 1930–40;
the top and bottom pairs are
particularly striking*

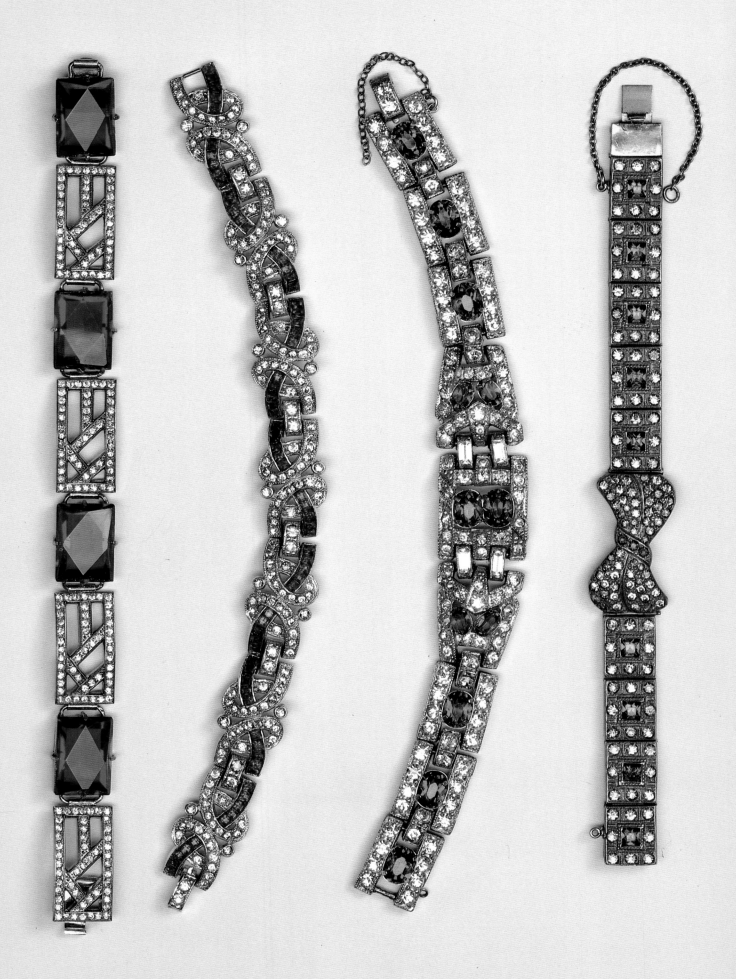

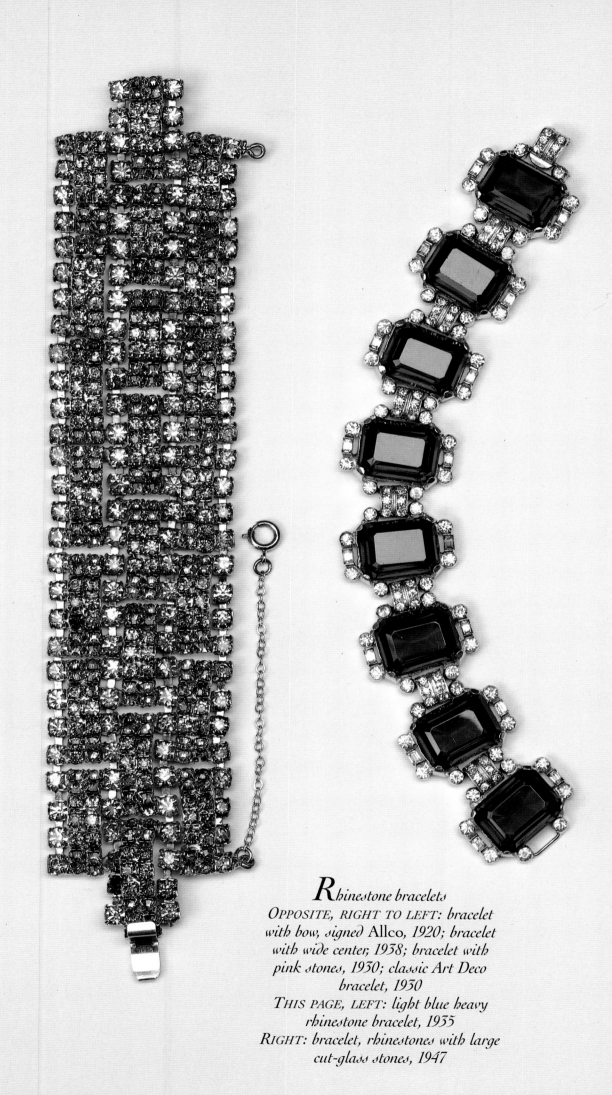

*R*hinestone bracelets

OPPOSITE, RIGHT TO LEFT: *bracelet with bow, signed Allco, 1920; bracelet with wide center, 1938; bracelet with pink stones, 1930; classic Art Deco bracelet, 1930*

THIS PAGE, LEFT: *light blue heavy rhinestone bracelet, 1935*

RIGHT: *bracelet, rhinestones with large cut-glass stones, 1947*

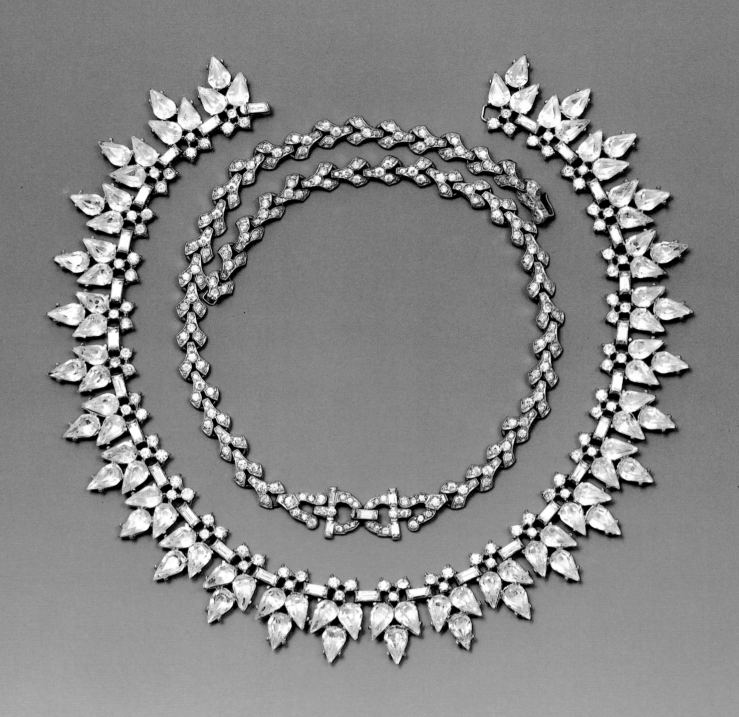

*Rhinestone necklaces set
with white stones
INSIDE: 1935
OUTSIDE: signed Trifari, 1940*

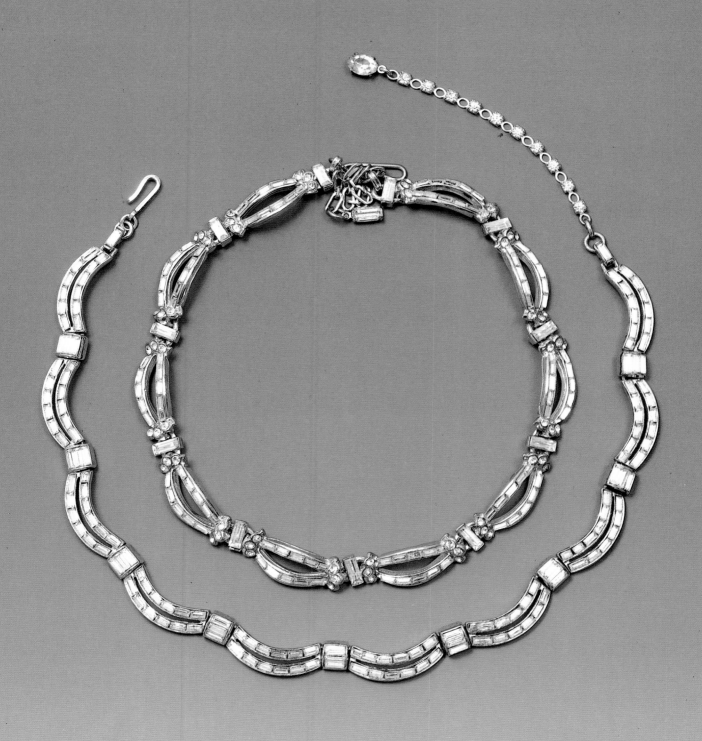

*Rhinestone necklaces in striking bowed
forms, set with baguette stones, both 1940*

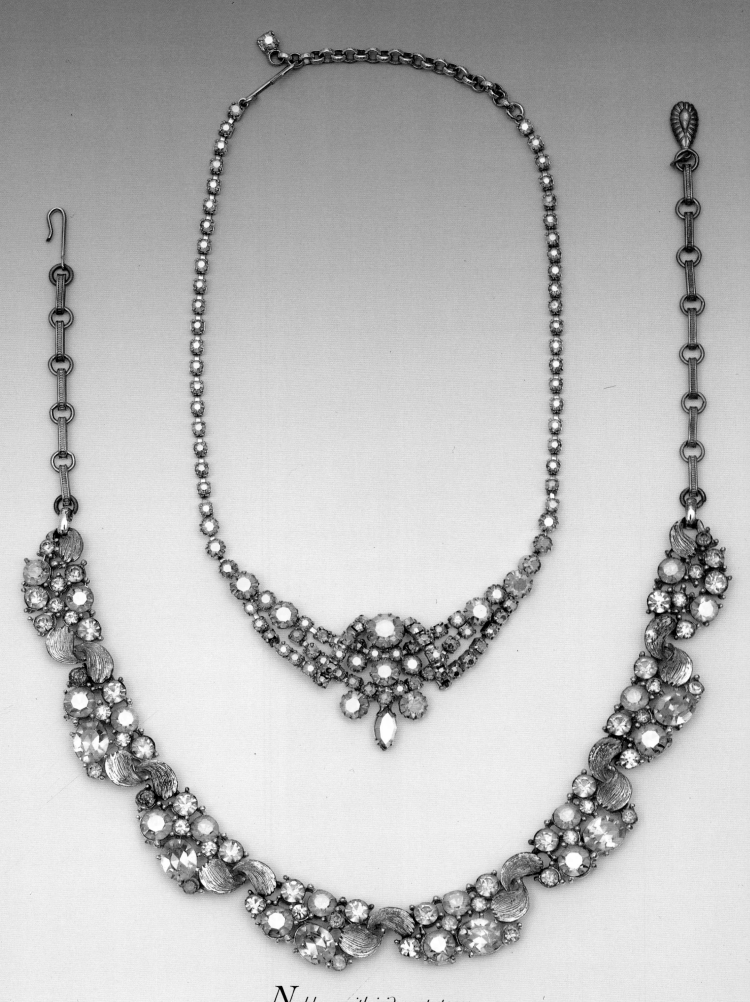

Necklaces with iridescent stones
INSIDE: *1940*
OUTSIDE: *signed Lisner, 1950*

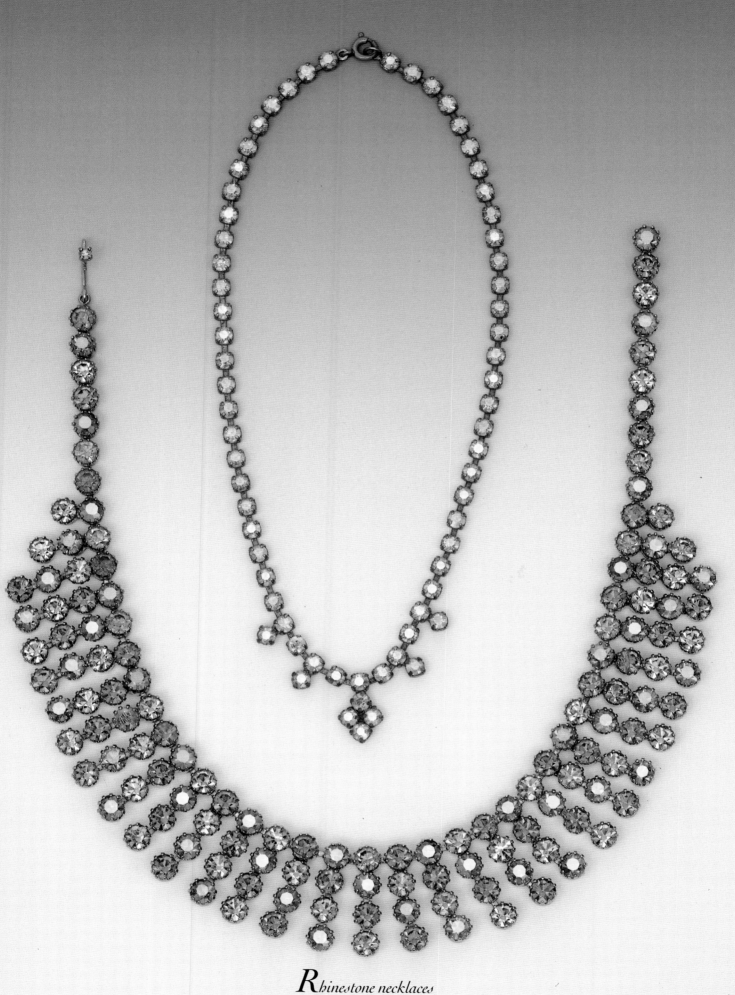

*R*hinestone necklaces
INSIDE: 1940
OUTSIDE: 1940

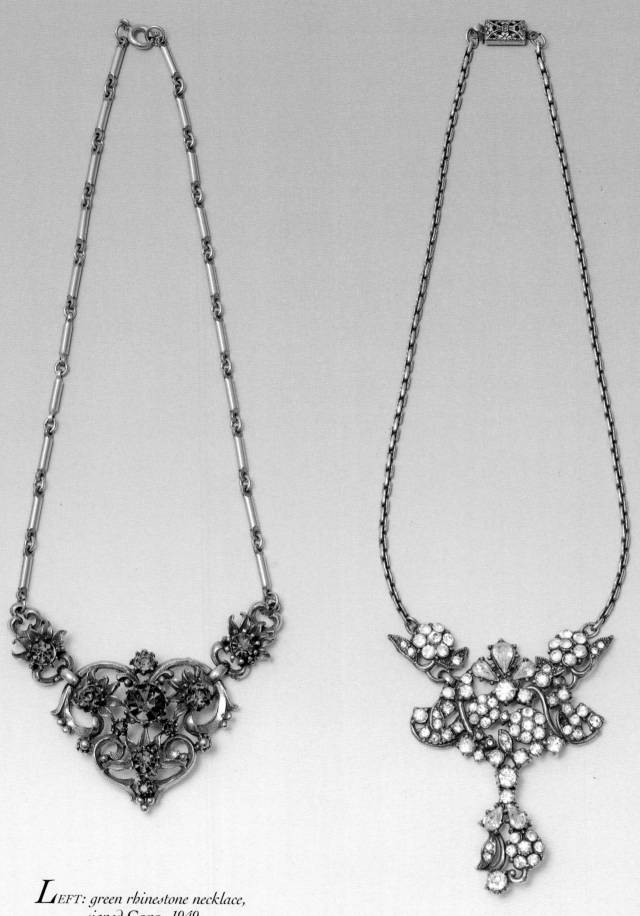

*L*EFT: *green rhinestone necklace,*
signed Coro, 1949
*R*IGHT: *Jugendstil necklace, white*
rhinestones on brass, 1920
*O*PPOSITE: *Art Deco necklaces*
*L*EFT: *rhinestones with topaz-colored*
pendant, 1930
*R*IGHT: *rhinestones with black glass, 1935*

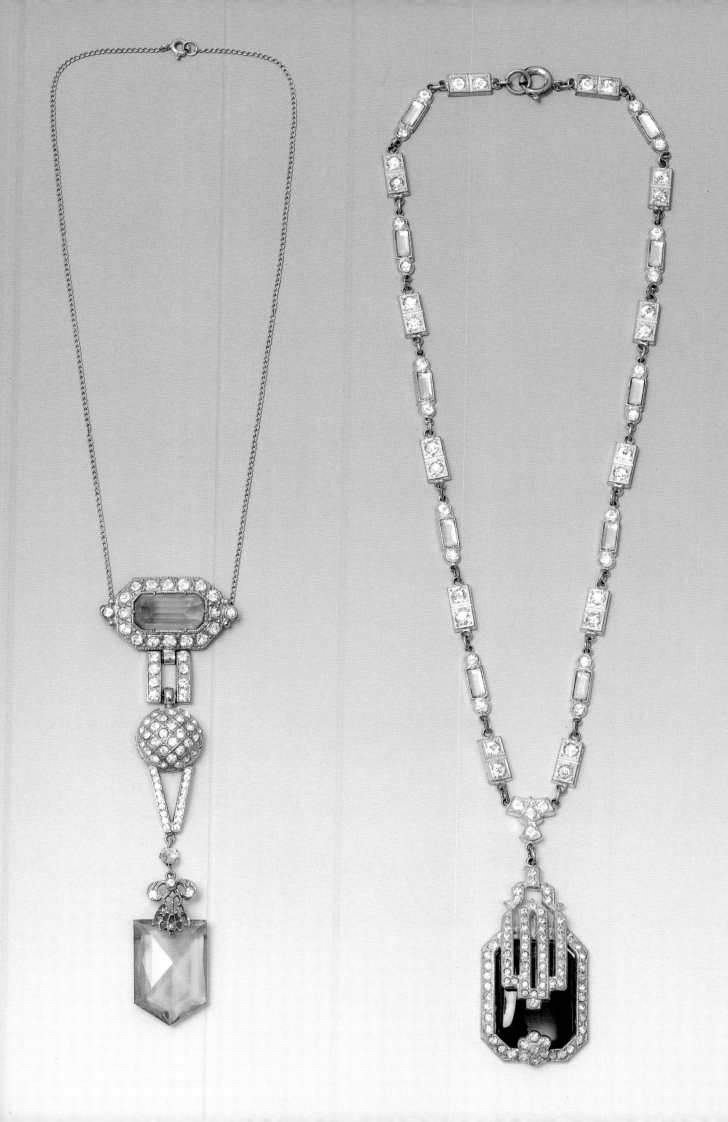

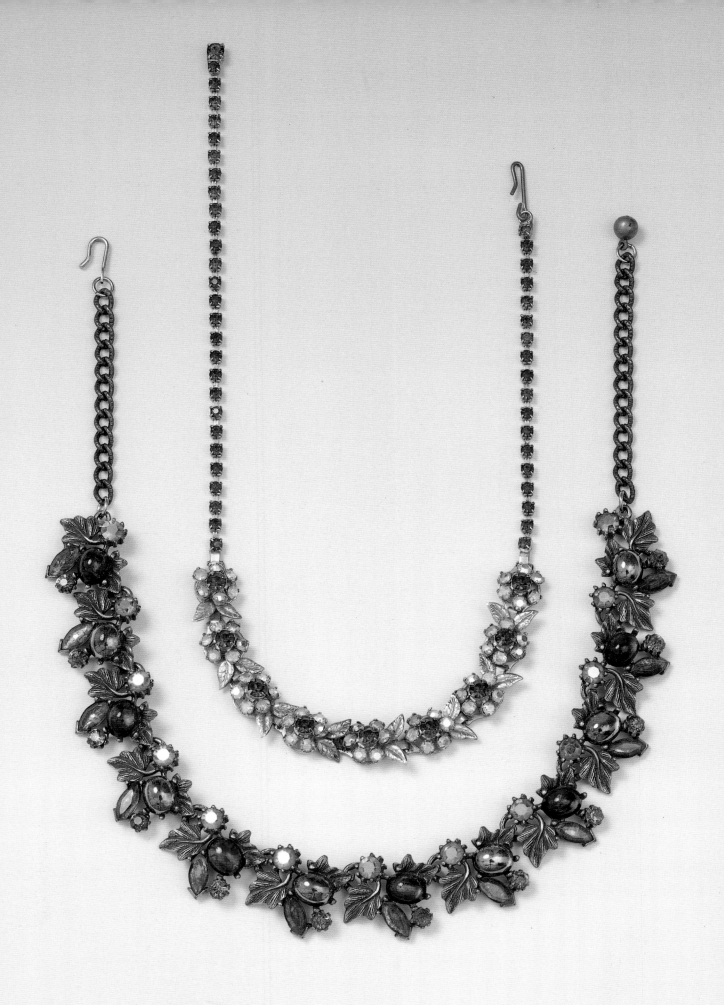

*F*loral rhinestone necklaces
INSIDE: 1940
OUTSIDE: 1945

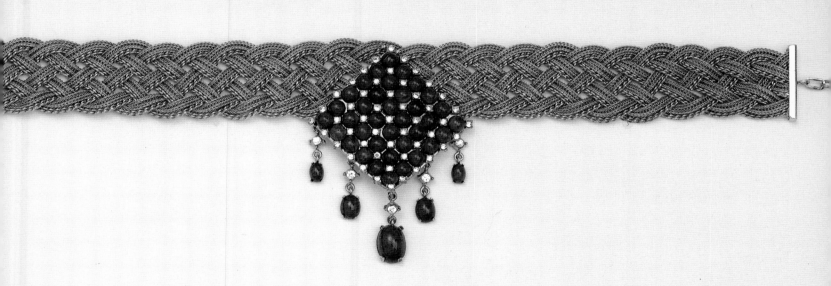

Necklace by Grossé, 1970

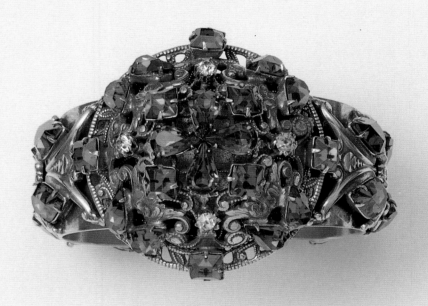

ABOVE: large bangle, 1940
OPPOSITE, TOP: bangle, 1930
BOTTOM: topaz-colored bangle, signed
Hobé, *1955*

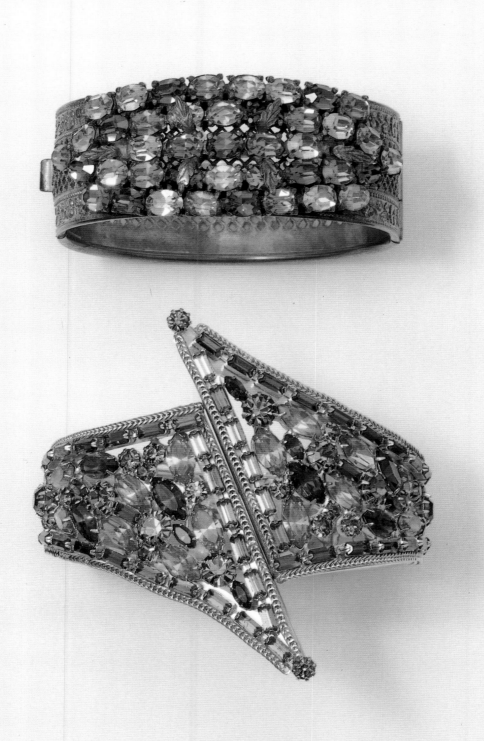

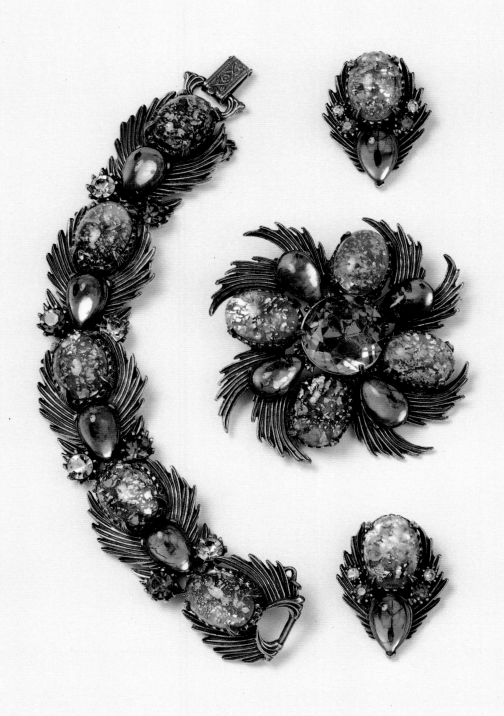

*Bracelet, brooch, and clip-on earrings
set, signed* Florenza, *1955*

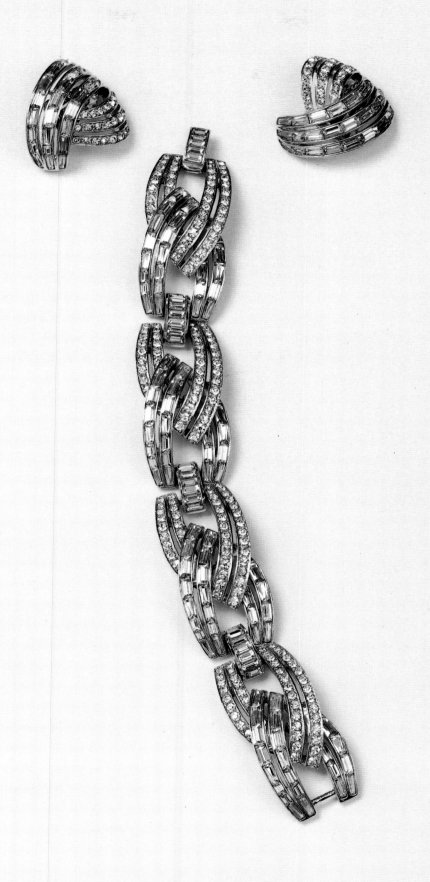

*Bracelet and clip-on earrings set, white
rhinestones, some baguette-cut, 1940*

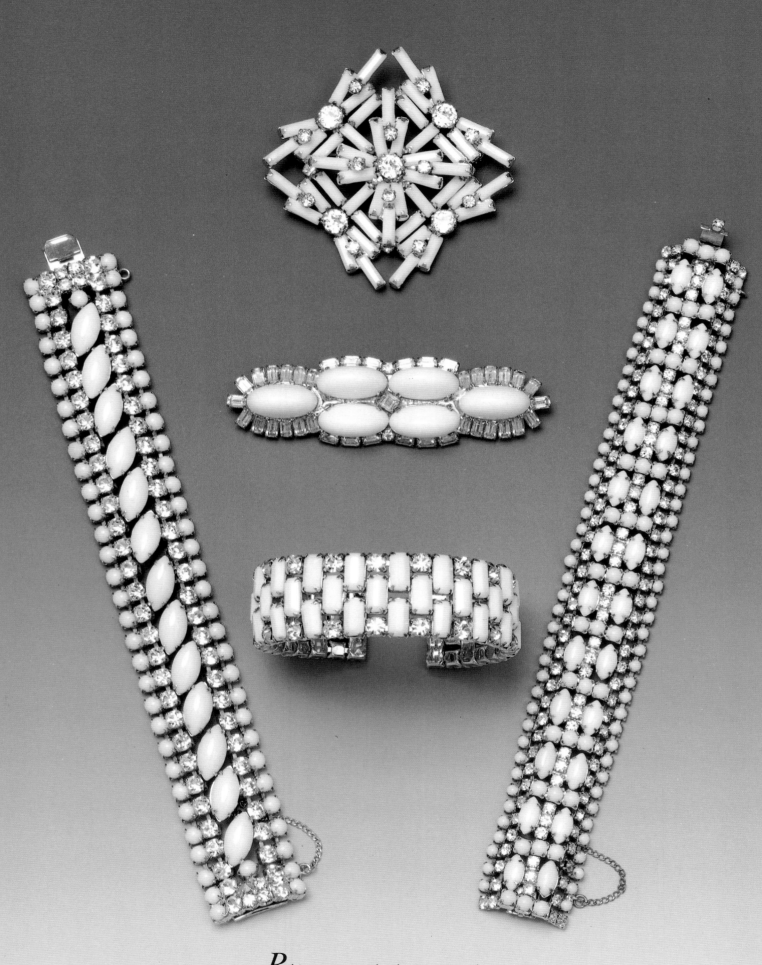

Rhinestones with white opaque glass
LEFT: *bracelet, signed* Weiss, *1955*
CENTER: *bracelet, signed* Weiss, *1955*
RIGHT: *bracelet, signed* Kramer of
New York, *1950*

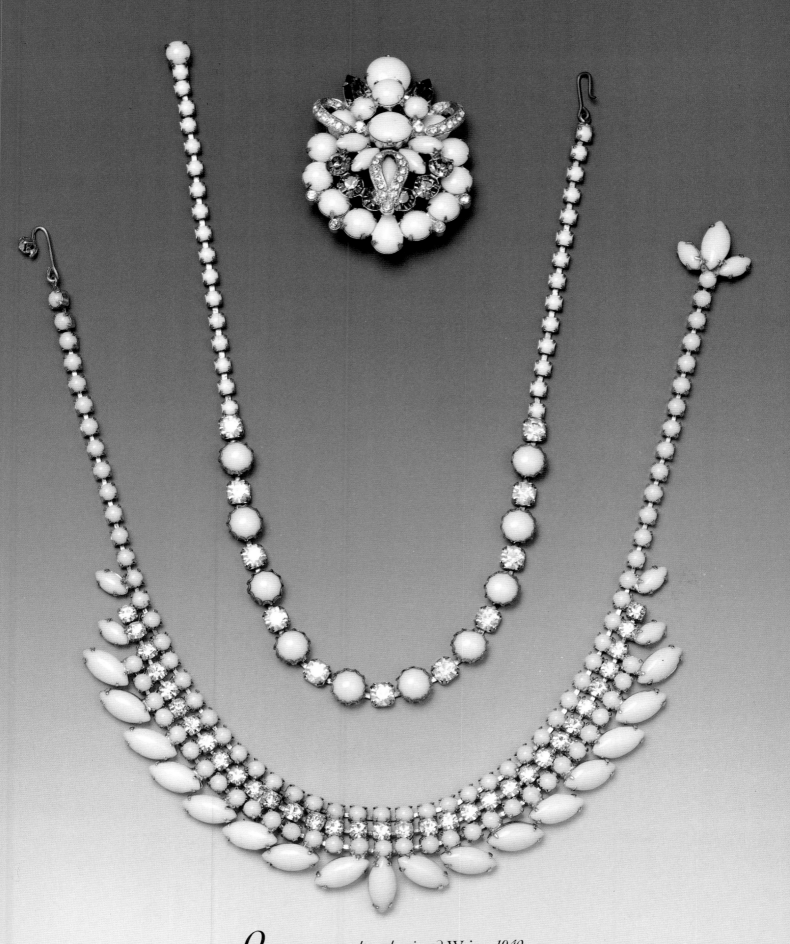

*O*PPOSITE, TOP: *brooch, signed* Weiss, *1940*
CENTER: *brooch, signed* De Lillo, *1950*
THIS PAGE, TOP: *brooch, signed*
Eisenberg Ice, *1955*
CENTER: *necklace, 1940*
BOTTOM: *necklace, signed* Weiss, *1955*

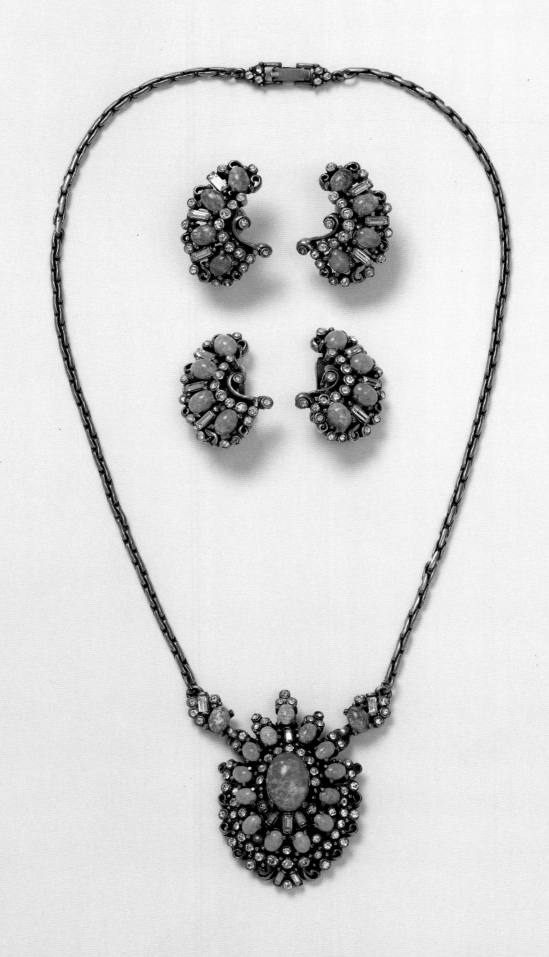

*S*et, necklace and two pairs of clip-on
earrings, opalescent rhinestones, signed
Hollycraft, 1955

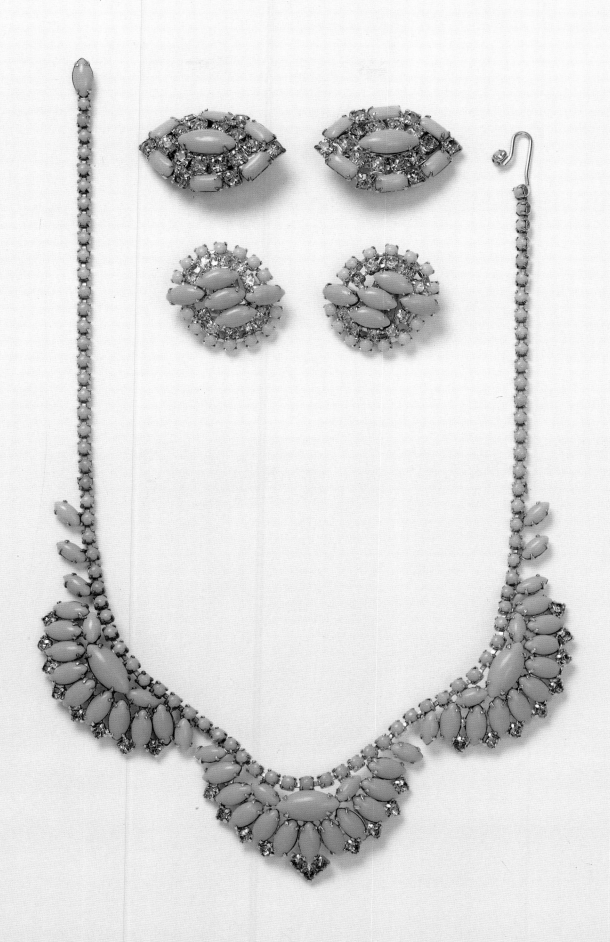

*S*et, necklace and two pairs of clip-on
earrings, white and blue rhinestones with
light blue glass stones, 1955

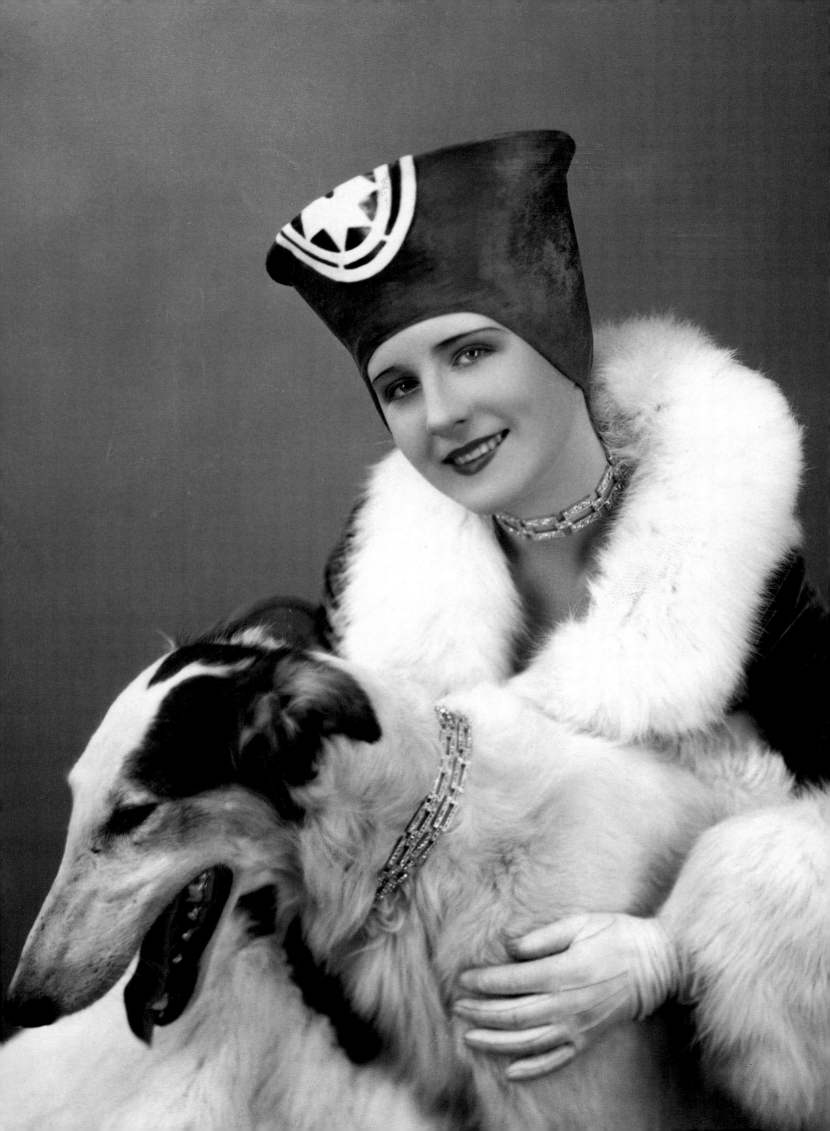

Animals

*S*omething stirring on the lapel: from cats and company to bugs, fish, and bumblebees — the prettiest specimens of the animal kingdom lounge, flutter, buzz, and crawl. Dressed up with shimmering stones, the aquatic element sends its most elegant messenger. And always there are butterflies, those timeless decorative darlings of fashion. The joyful feeling of utter weightlessness, captured in rhinestones.

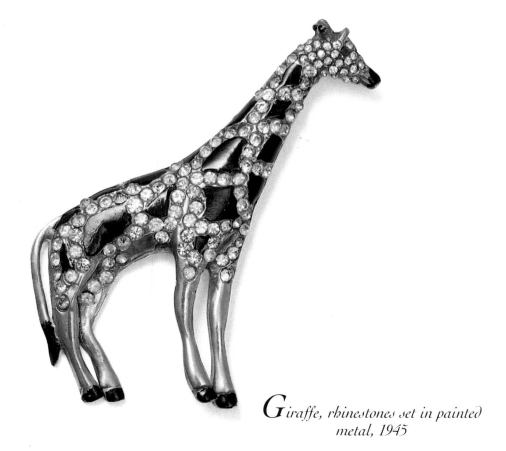

Giraffe, rhinestones set in painted metal, 1945

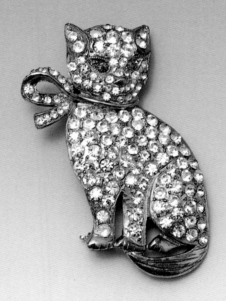

ABOVE: *cat with bow, white
rhinestones, 1935*
OPPOSITE, LEFT TO RIGHT: *rhinestone
terrier, 1940; rhinestone poodle, 1940;
rhinestone dog, 1960*

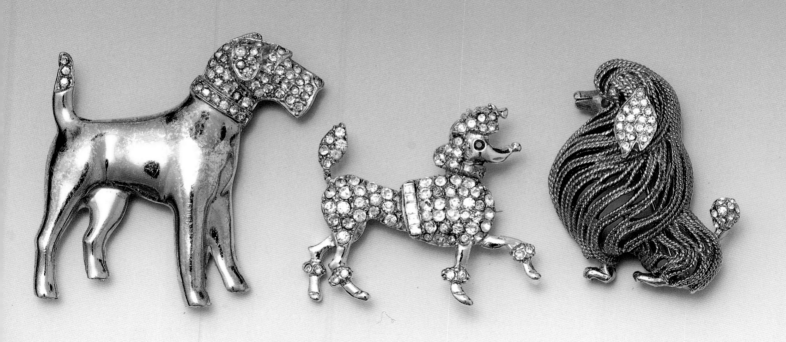

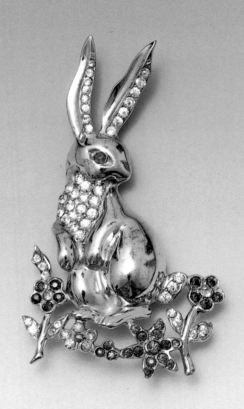

*H*are with flowers, rhinestones on
partially painted metal, 1940

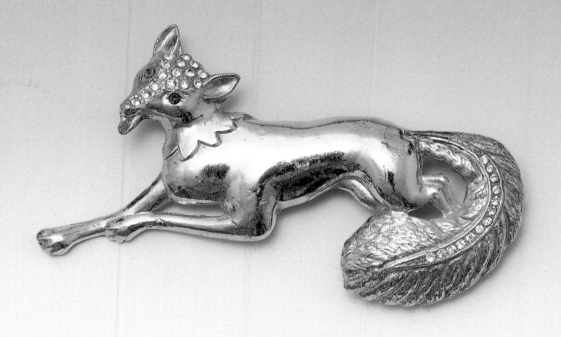

Fox set with rhinestones, 1938

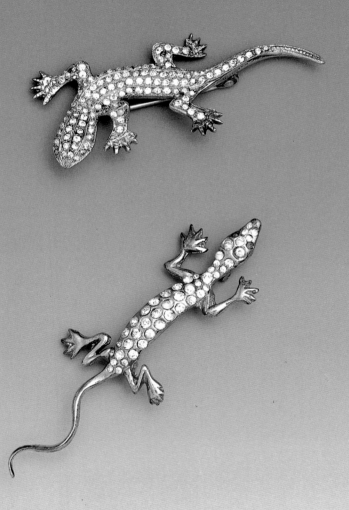

Lizard pins, all 1920

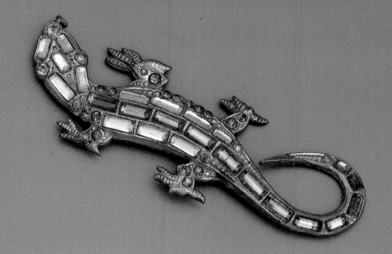

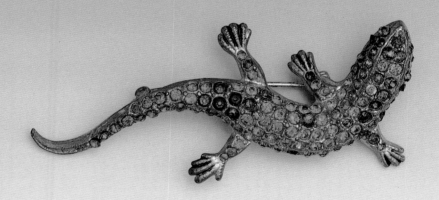

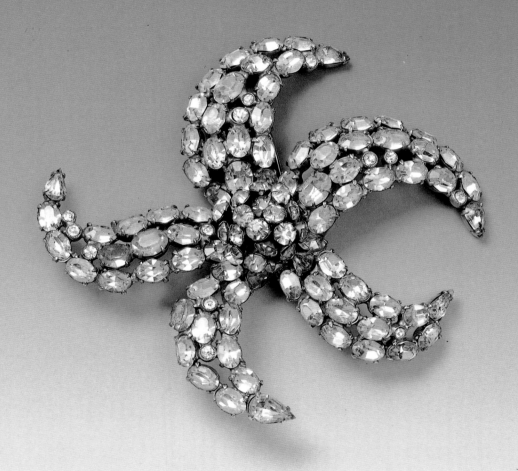

*White rhinestone starfish, clothing
clip, signed* HC, *1920*

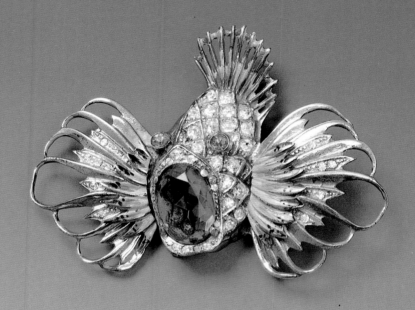

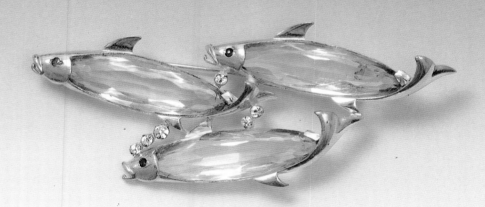

*T*OP: *Siamese fighting fish, rhinestones
on gold-colored silver, signed* Coro, *1940*
*B*OTTOM: *three coral-colored fish, brooch,
rhinestones with plastic, 1940*

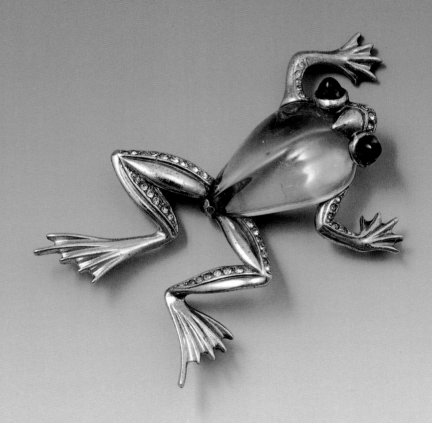

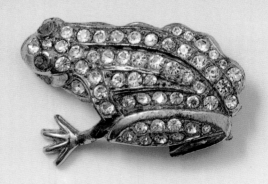

*T*OP: *frog, rhinestones with acrylic,
signed* Trifari, *1950*
*B*OTTOM: *frog with white
rhinestones, 1950*

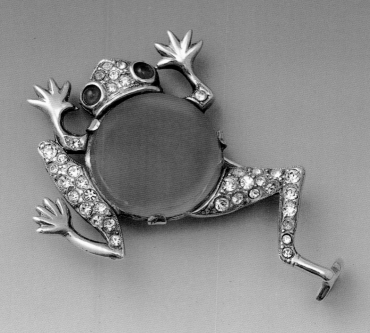

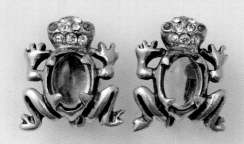

*T*OP: *frog with red glass eyes, agate body, and rhinestones on gold-colored silver; 1940*
*B*OTTOM: *frog earrings, rhinestones on gold-colored silver; 1940*

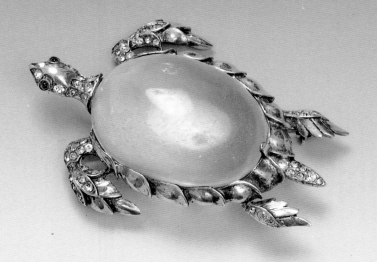

Swimming sea turtle, rhinestones with acrylic, signed Trifari, *1940*

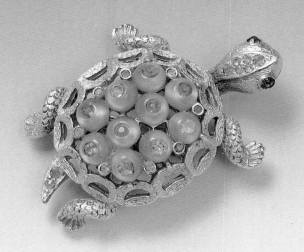

*Sea turtle, rhinestones with pink
pearls, 1960*

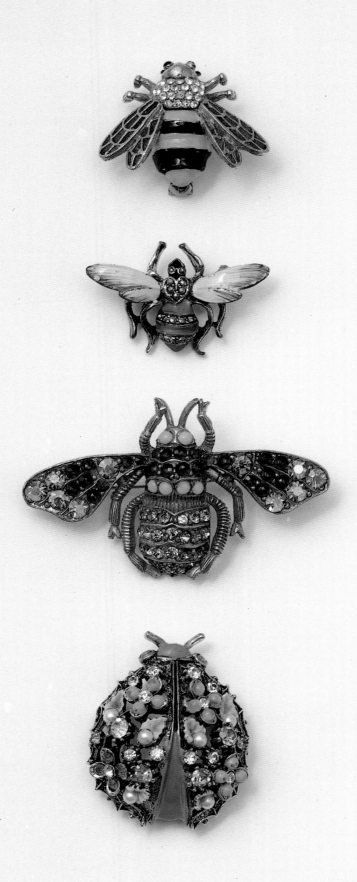

Rhinestone fly and beetle pins, 1935–48

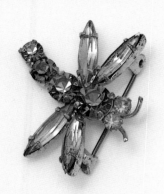

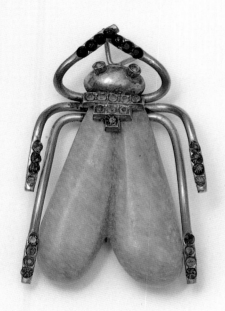

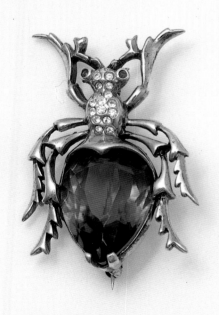

*T*OP: *rhinestone fly, 1950*
CENTER: *beetle, rhinestones and green*
Bakelite, 1938
BOTTOM: *Stag beetle, rhinestones on*
gold-colored silver, 1940

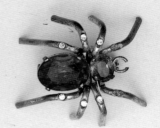

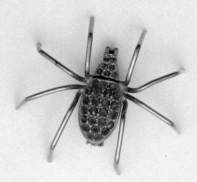

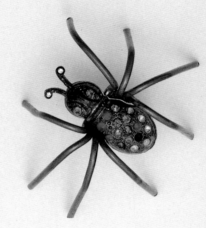

*S*pider pins, white and colored
rhinestones on painted metal, 1930–40

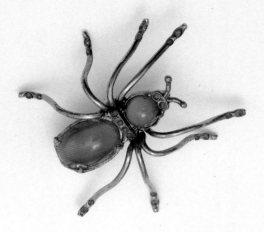

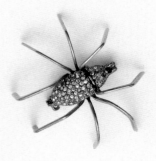

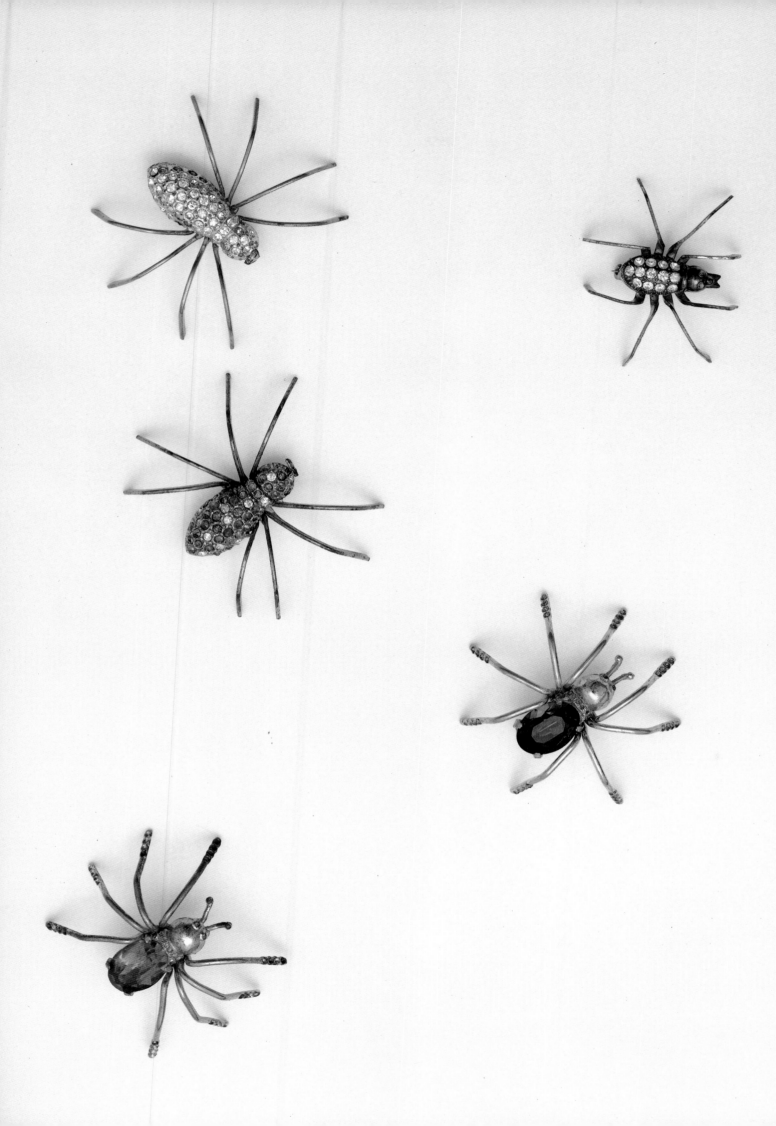

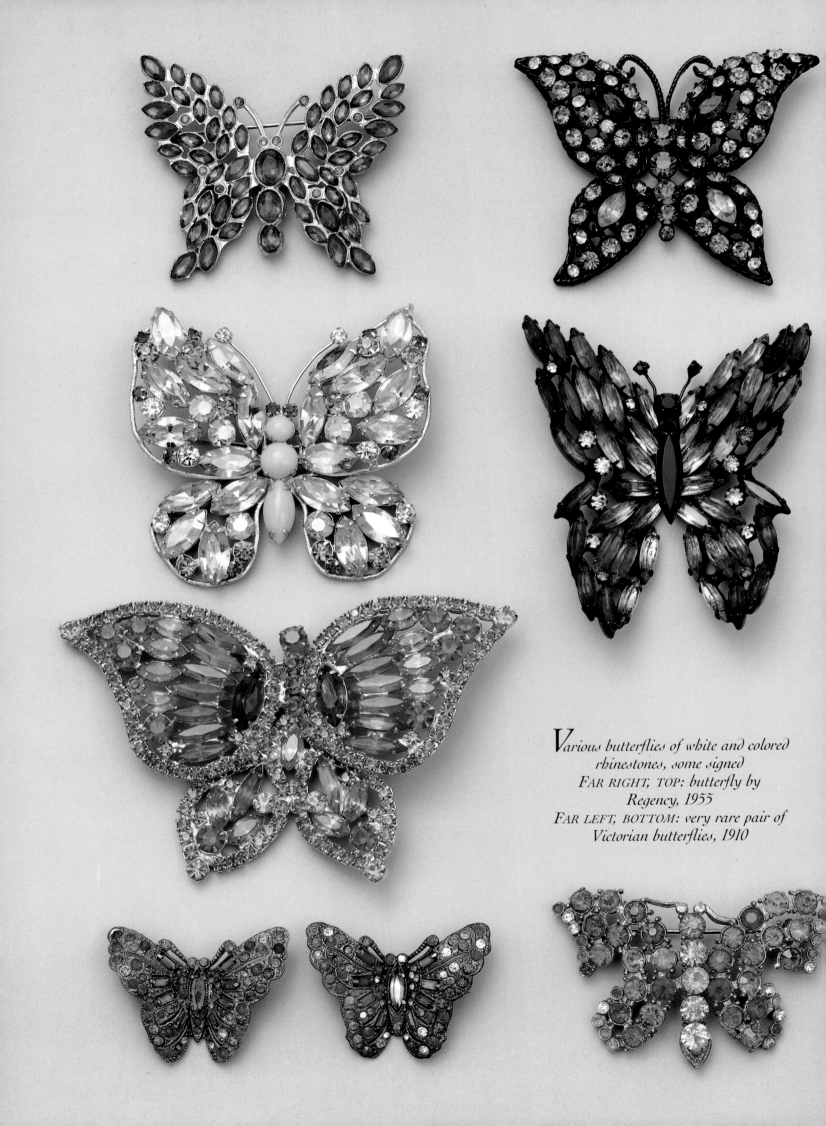

Various butterflies of white and colored rhinestones, some signed
FAR RIGHT, TOP: *butterfly by Regency, 1955*
FAR LEFT, BOTTOM: *very rare pair of Victorian butterflies, 1910*

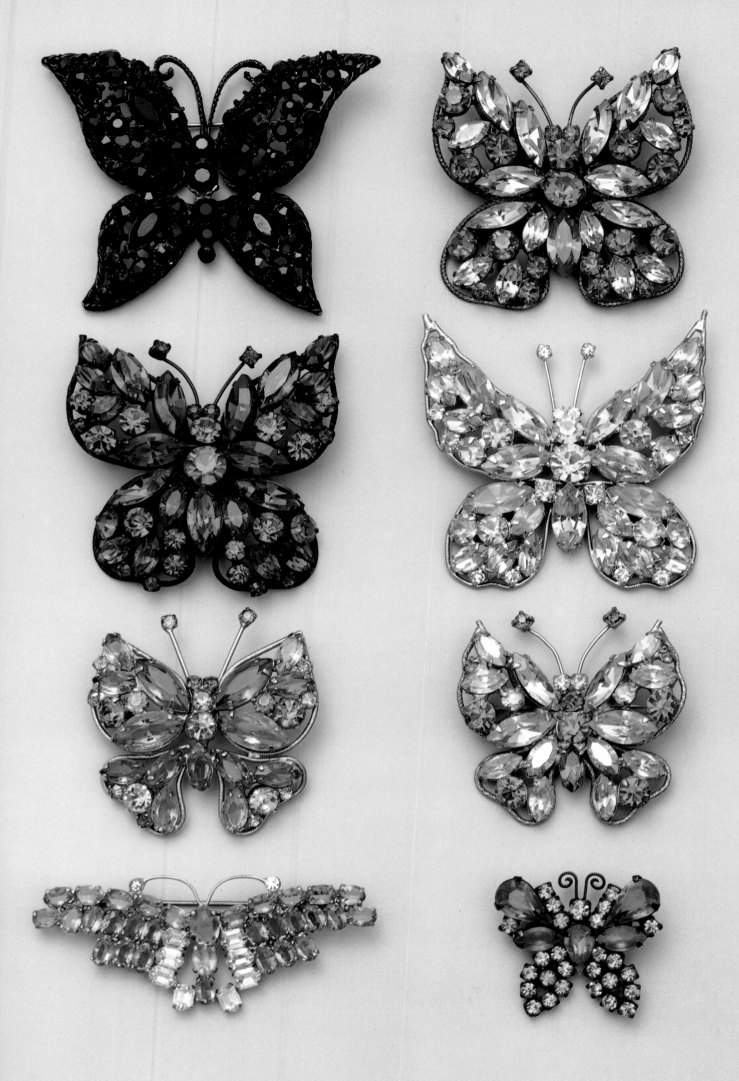

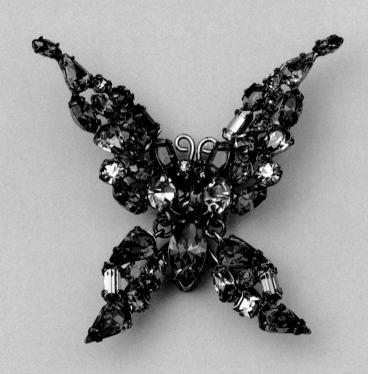

Butterfly pin with movable wings,
known as a trembler, 1955

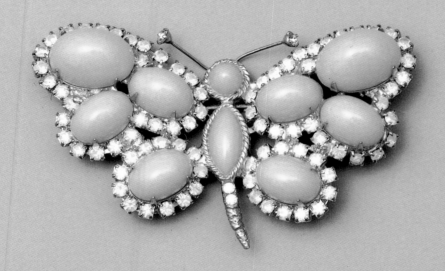

*Large butterfly pin, opalescent
rhinestones with yellow glass cabochons,
1955*

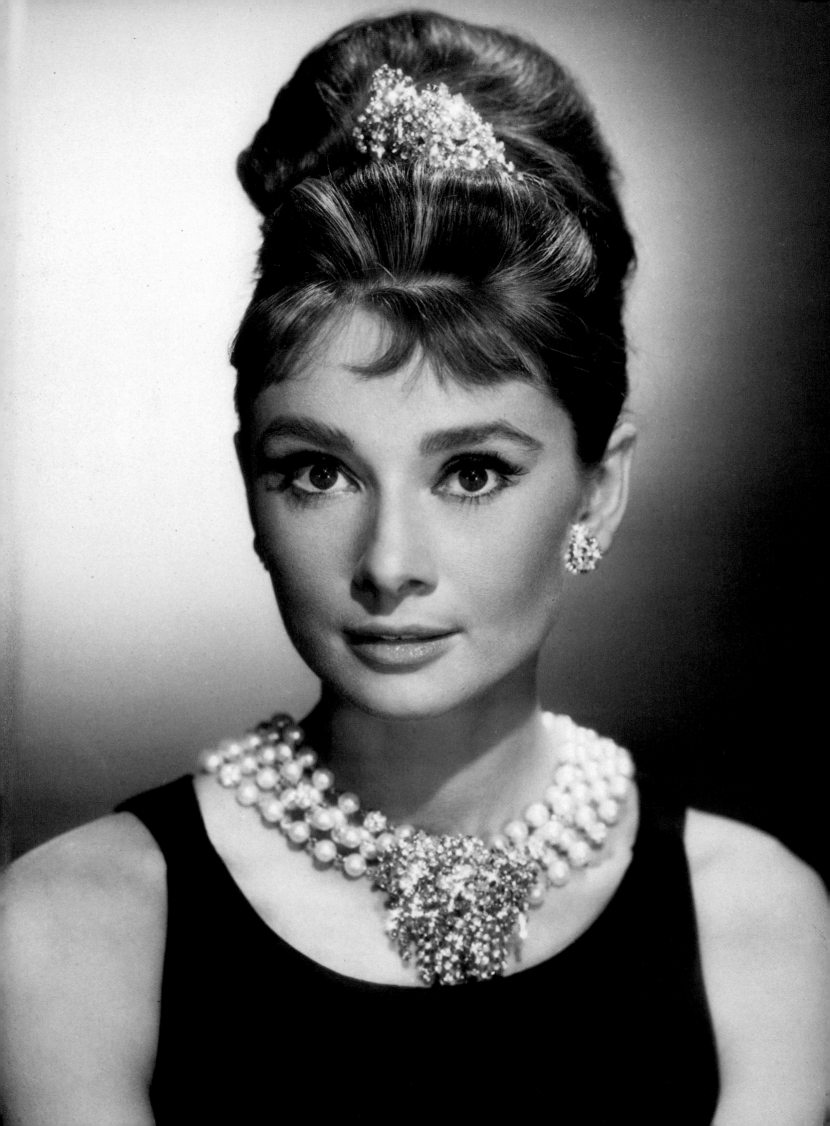

Eisenberg

Somewhere over the rainbow . . ." Somewhere between the day and the dream lies great fortune, as for Audrey Hepburn in her most beguiling role. *Breakfast at Tiffany's*, with hot coffee in paper cups and little sighs on the way home. Holly Golightly will never marry a rich prince; rather, a humble writer who gives her a shiny tin ring. Perhaps a piece by Eisenberg, America's greatest master of the rhinestone. The shine and color of his rare creations rival the most precious of stones. They give to rhinestone jewelry a magnificent new look and to every woman the feeling of being as regal as a princess.

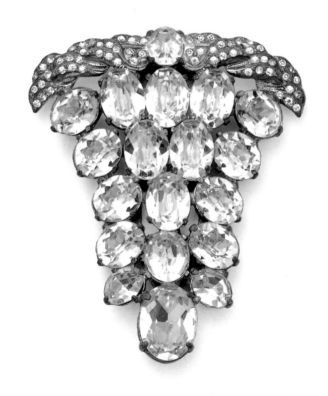

Clothing clip, signed Eisenberg Original, *1935, actual size*

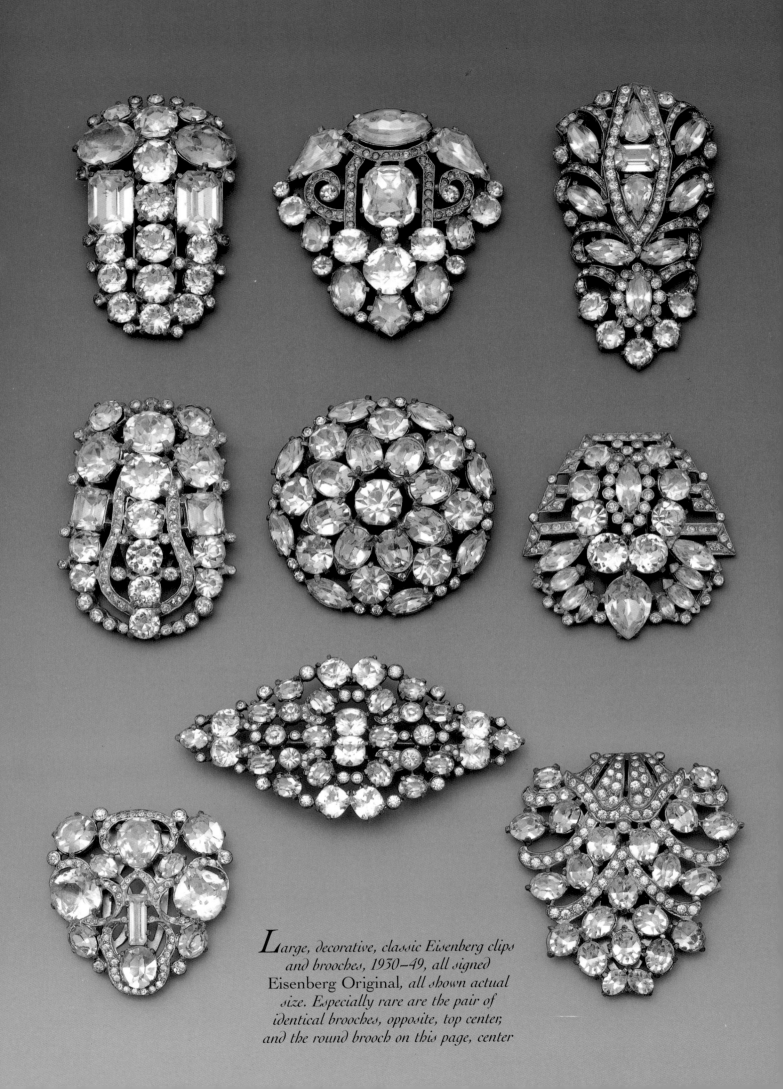

Large, decorative, classic Eisenberg clips and brooches, 1930–49, all signed Eisenberg Original, *all shown actual size. Especially rare are the pair of identical brooches, opposite, top center, and the round brooch on this page, center*

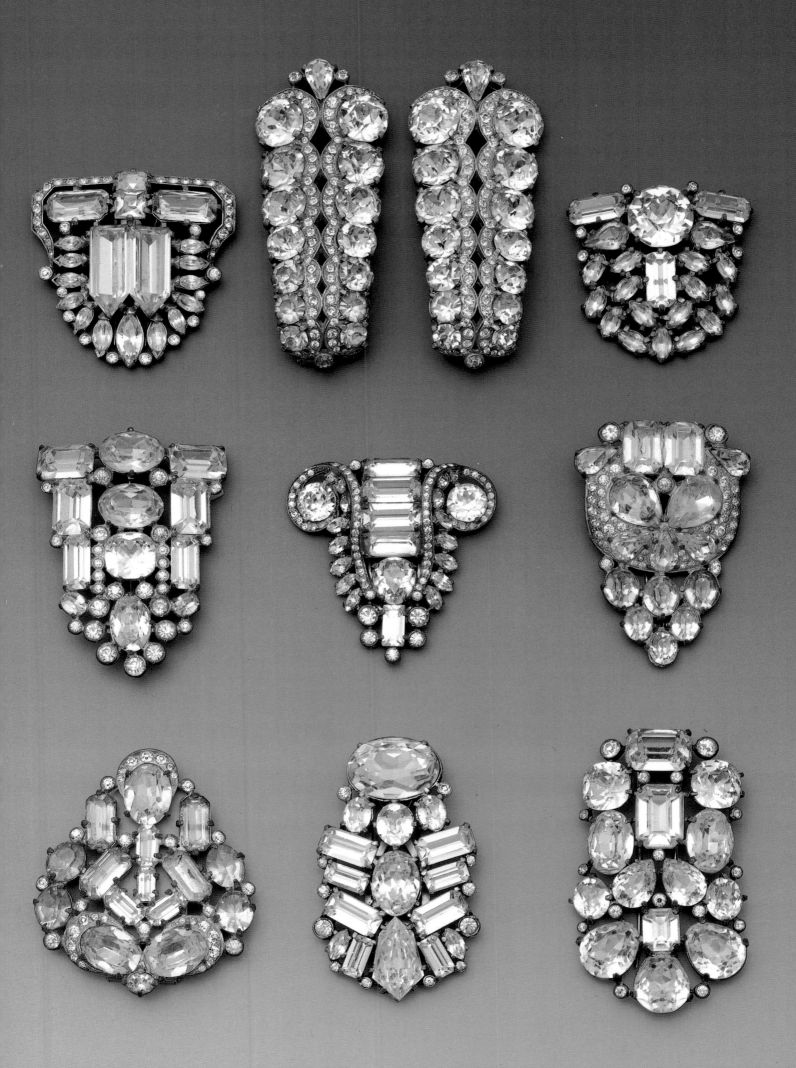

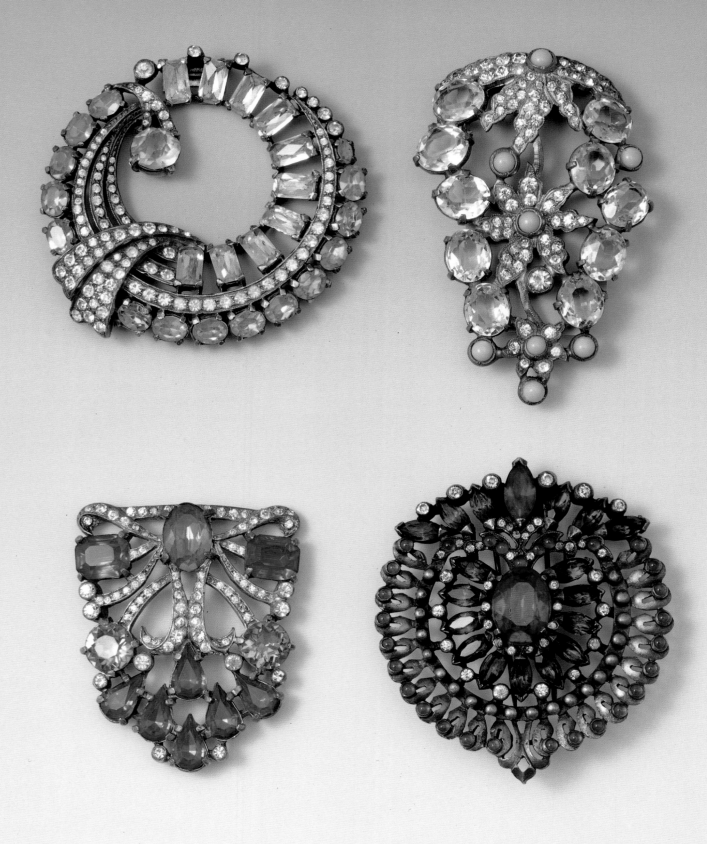

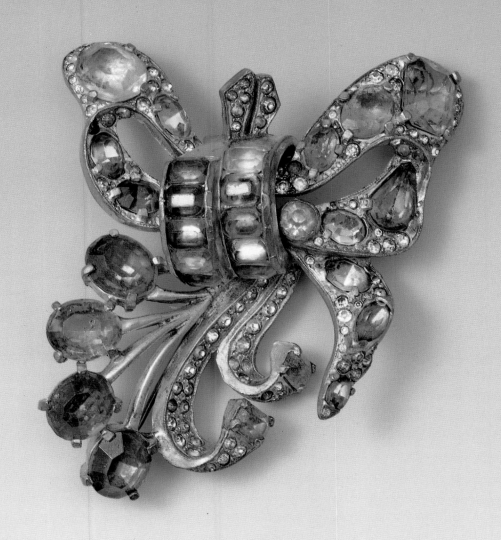

Opposite: brooches, signed Eisenberg
Original, 1940, slightly enlarged
ABOVE: bow brooch, signed Eisenberg
Original, 1940, slightly enlarged

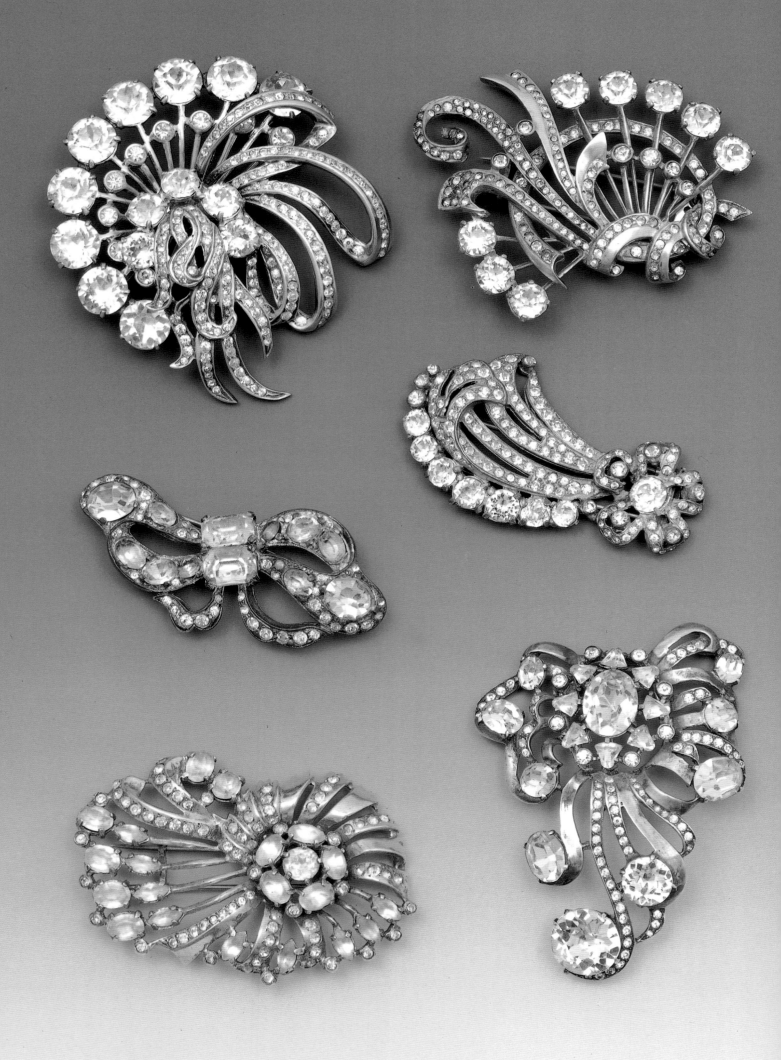

Decorative Eisenberg brooches and fur clips, all signed Eisenberg Original, *1920–40, except opposite, top left: brooch of rhodium-plated metal, signed* E, *1950*

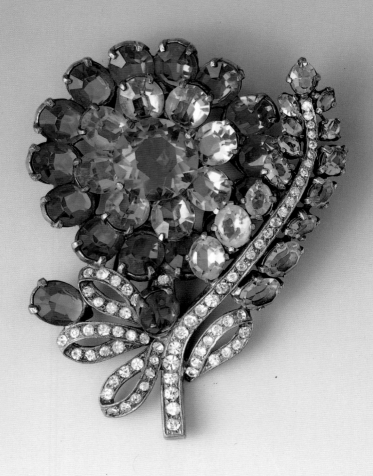

Large flower brooch, signed Eisenberg
Original, *1940, slightly enlarged*

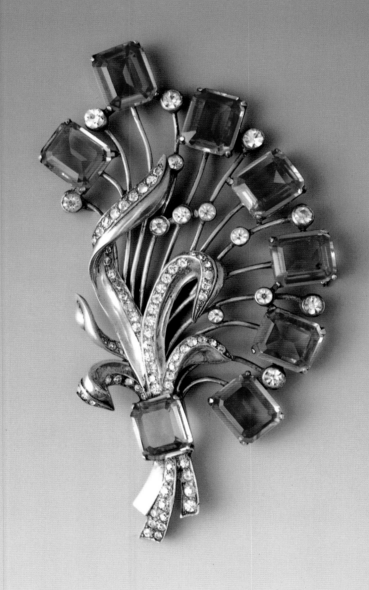

*R*are brooch with pink stones as
flowers, signed Eisenberg Original,
1940, slightly enlarged

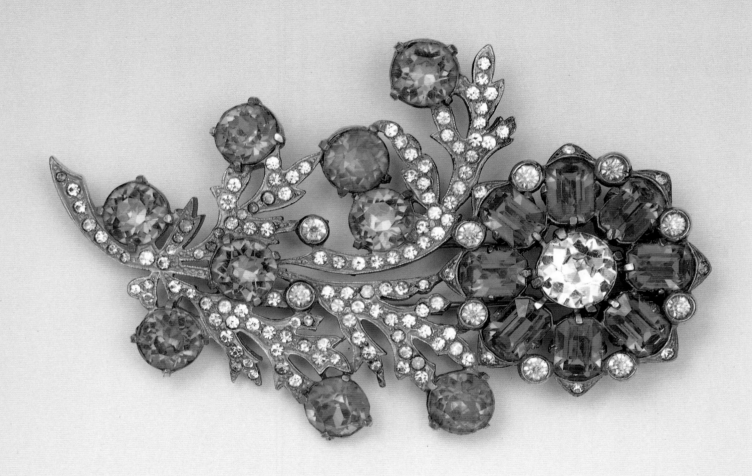

ABOVE: floral spray, signed Eisenberg
Original, *1940, slightly enlarged*
OPPOSITE: floral spray brooch with
flower buds, signed Eisenberg
Original, *1943, slightly enlarged*

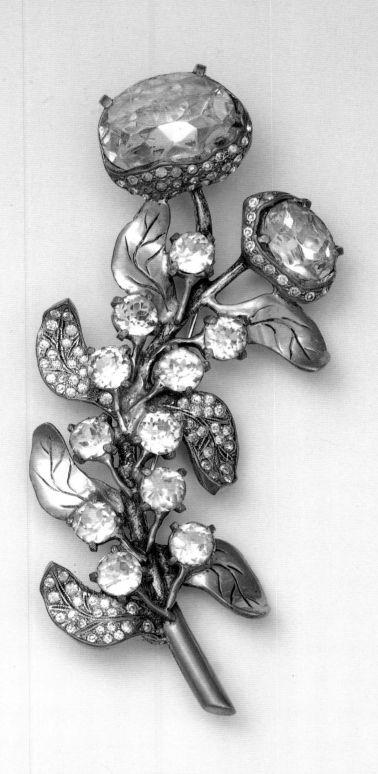

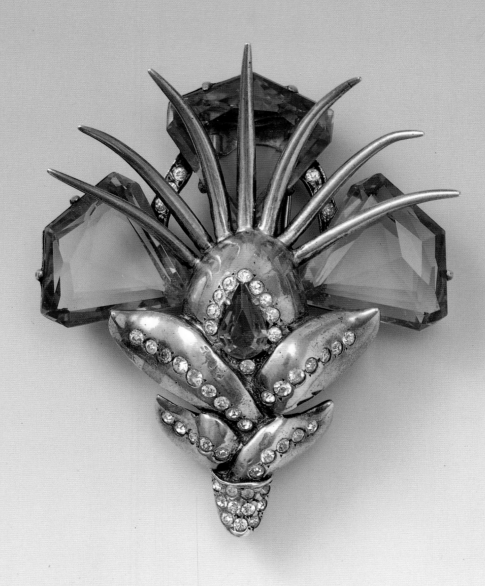

*ABOVE: fan-shaped floral brooch,
signed* Eisenberg Original, *1945,
slightly enlarged*
OPPOSITE: rare necklace, signed
Eisenberg Original, *with
complementary brooch, 1945,
slightly enlarged*

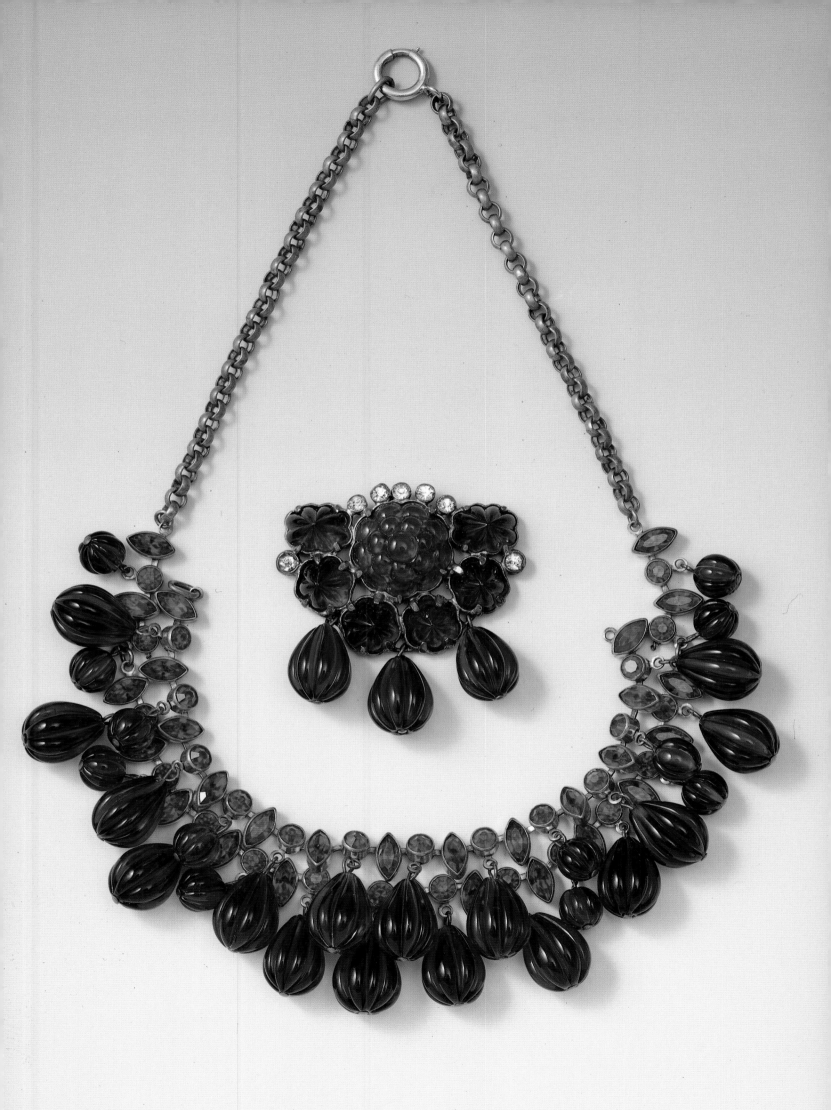

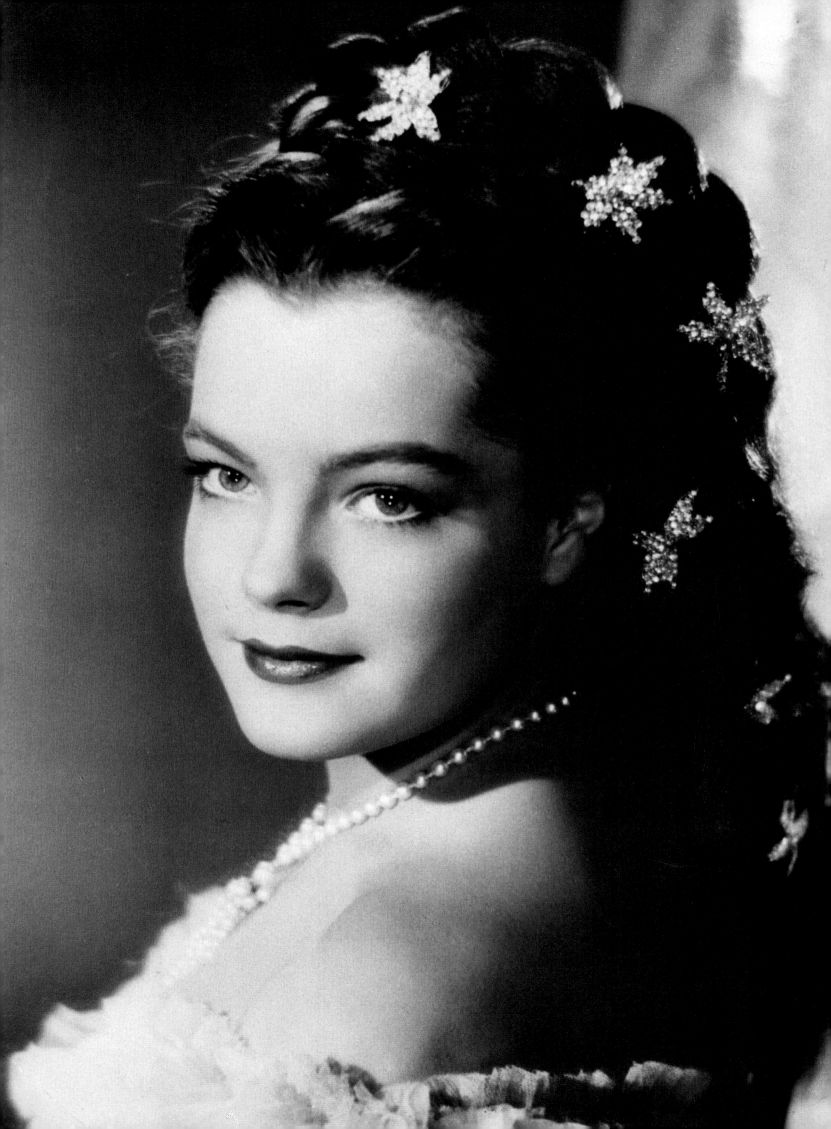

Stars

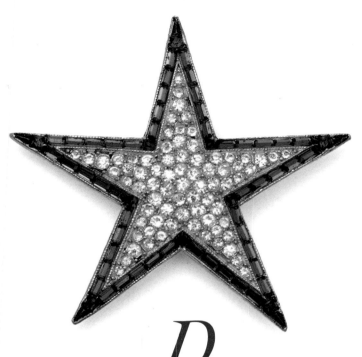

*D*o you know how many little stars there are?" In the richly braided hair of Empress Sissi almost as many stars twinkle as in the firmament itself. Of course, a real empress would wear only the prettiest diamonds. But for the young Romy Schneider rhinestones glitter just as beautifully. Old rhinestone stars today are a real godsend and especially cherished by their fans, because in the days of the empire and kings these heavenly pieces were seldom made, certainly out of respect for the originals, which were reserved as jewelry and medals for the honorable members of the royal house. Modern designers have rediscovered this graceful jewelry form for all hours of the day — giving it a genuinely stellar career.

Star brooch, white rhinestones with colored baguette-cut rhinestones, 1935

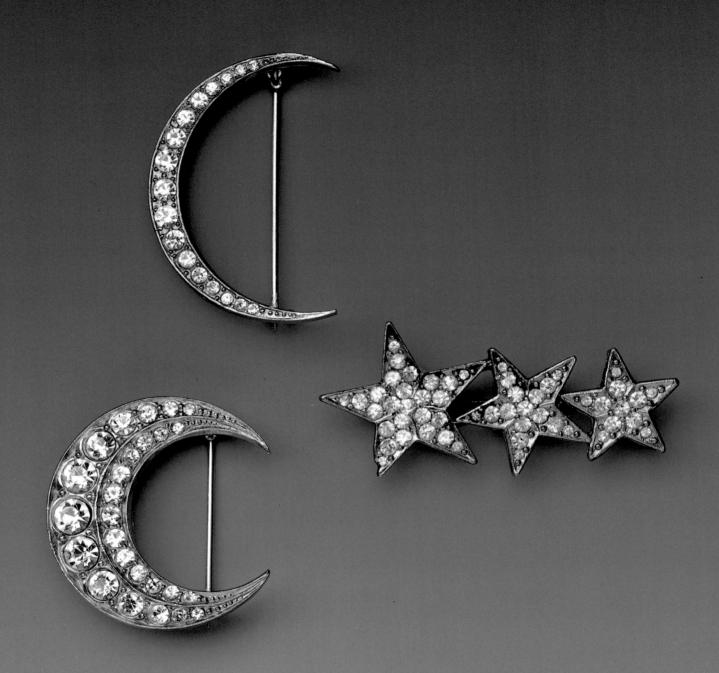

*ABOVE: stars and two crescent moon
brooches, white rhinestones on metal, all 1935
OPPOSITE: rare rhinestone star brooch
with large central round white stone, 1900*

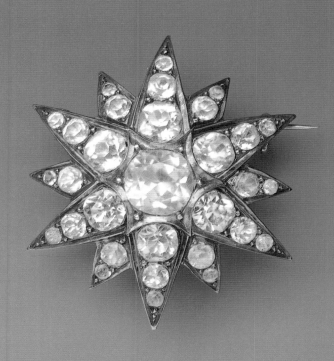

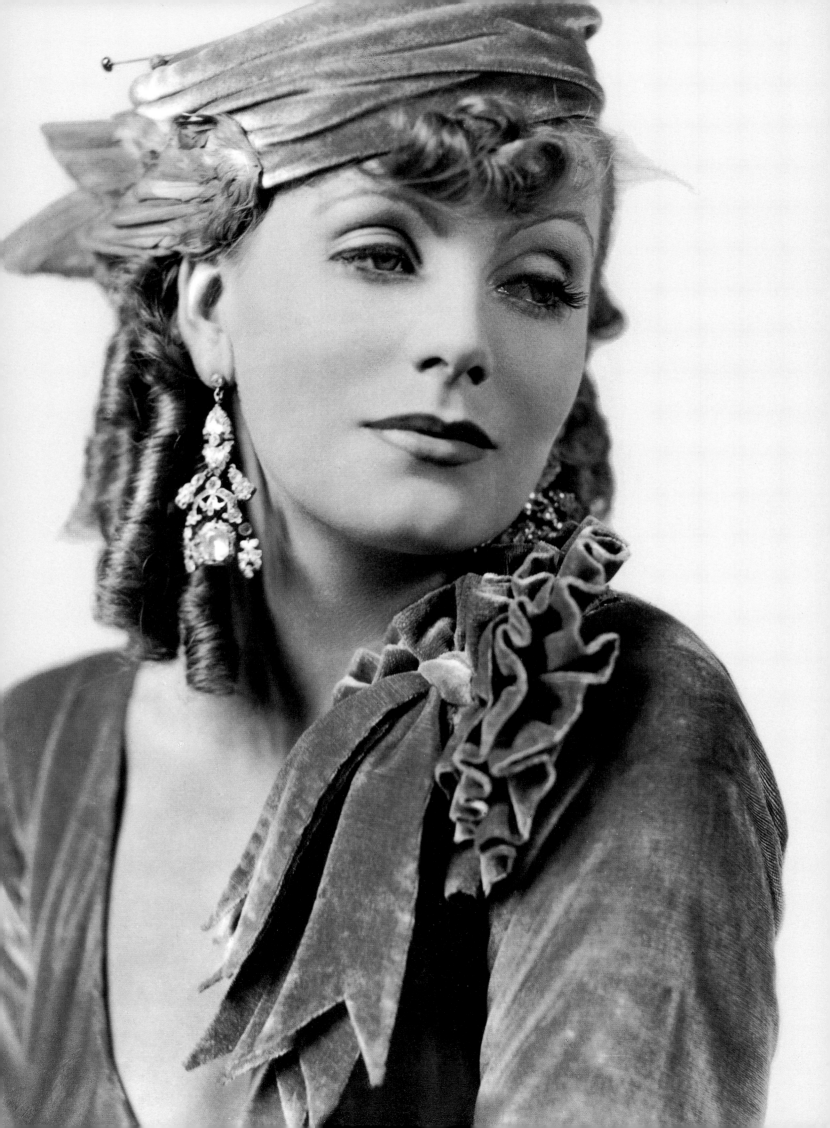

Earrings

*T*he earlobe seems to have been destined for beautiful jewelry. Dainty studs, lovely clips accentuate it with an individual touch; heavy drops and whole cascades of tiny rhinestones shimmer in all colors and swing with every little movement. Magnificent earrings in the rococo style ordered by Madame Pompadour and Madame Du Barry from Georges Frédéric Stras shone in the court. Today the motto is: The longer, the lovelier; the more extravagant, the better. And the styles that found favor with Greta Garbo and other legendary film stars also came to adorn the ears of many off-screen beauties. Because no other jewelry is as fascinatingly feminine and ever-new.

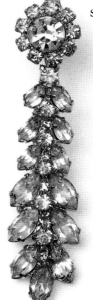
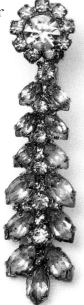

*W*hite rhinestone earrings, signed
Weiss, *1950*

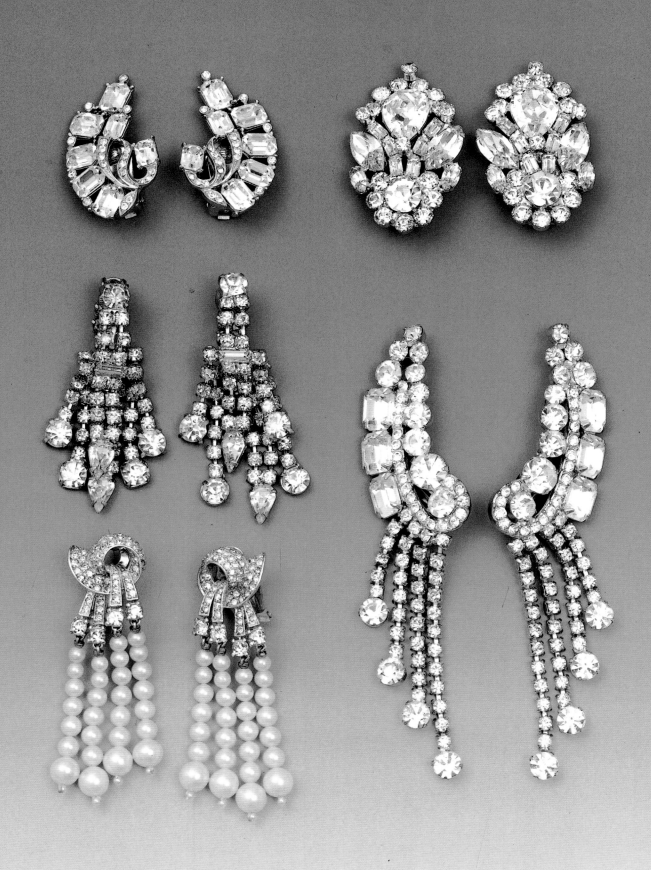

*E*arrings, 1940–55
CENTER, LEFT: *interesting double drop, 1940*
BOTTOM, LEFT: *hung with pearls and
signed* Pennino, *1940*

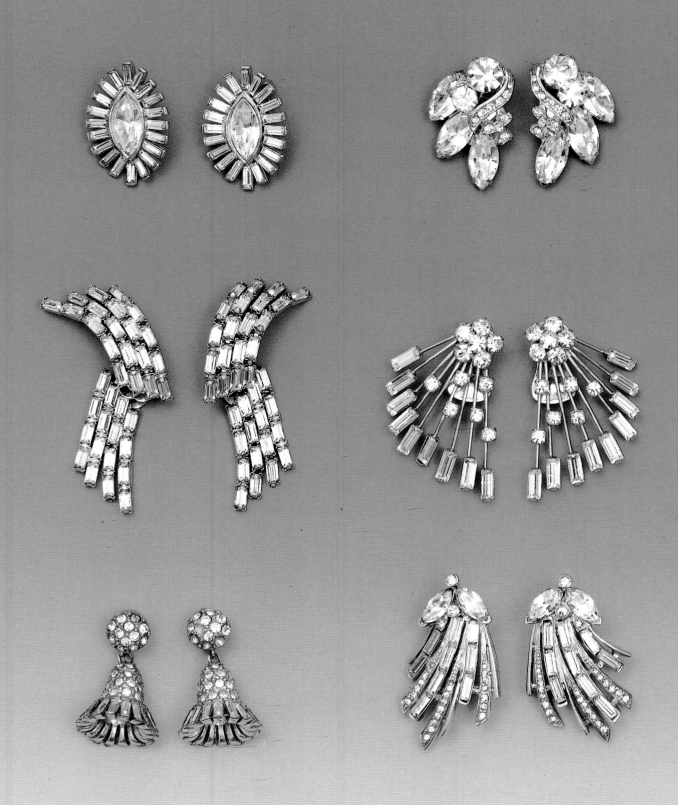

Clip-on earrings and studs, 1940–50
BOTTOM, RIGHT: *signed* Ora, 1940

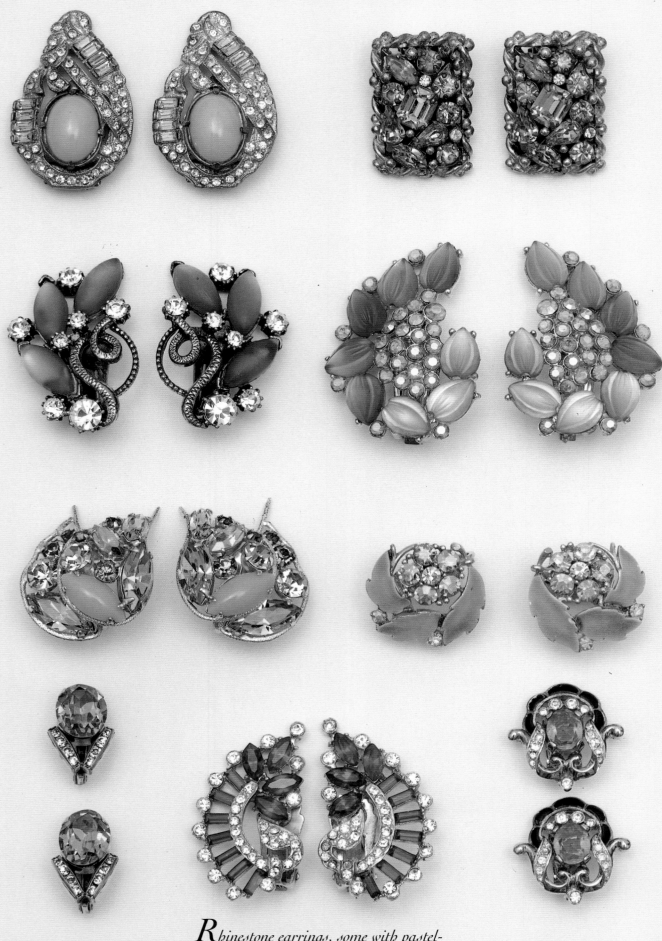

Rhinestone earrings, some with pastel-colored glass, 1930–50
TOP, LEFT: *Art Deco clip-on earrings, 1935*
TOP, RIGHT: *signed* Hollycraft, *1950*
BOTTOM, LEFT: *German rhinestone clip-on earrings, 1930*

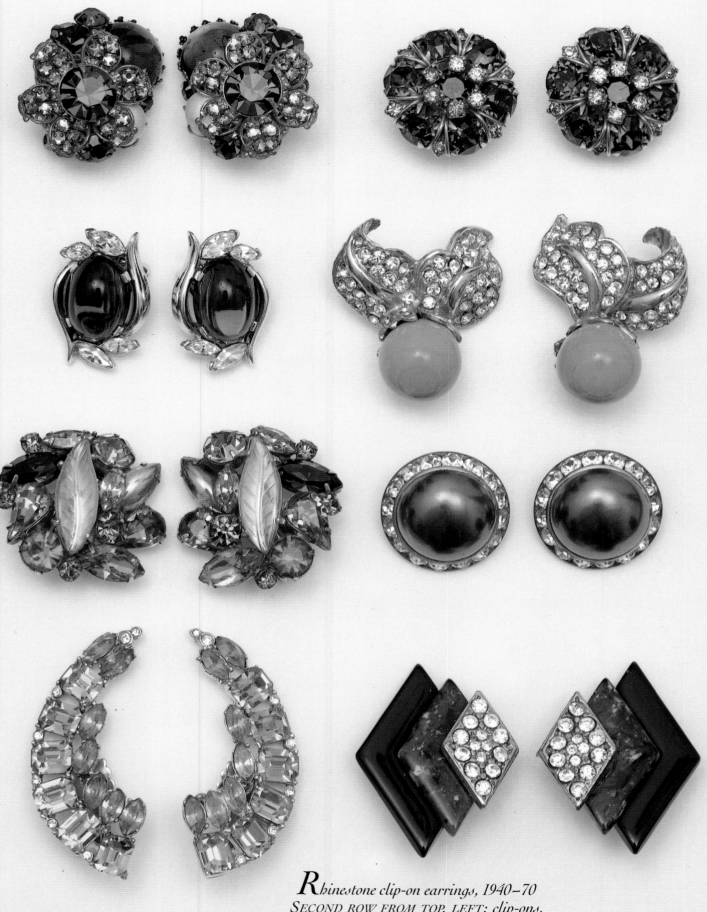

Rhinestone clip-on earrings, 1940–70
SECOND ROW FROM TOP, LEFT: *clip-ons,
signed* Trifari, *1955*
SECOND ROW FROM TOP, RIGHT: *clip-
ons, signed* Kenneth Lane, *1960*
BOTTOM ROW, LEFT: *clip-on
earrings, 1940*
BOTTOM ROW, RIGHT: *clip-ons, 1970*

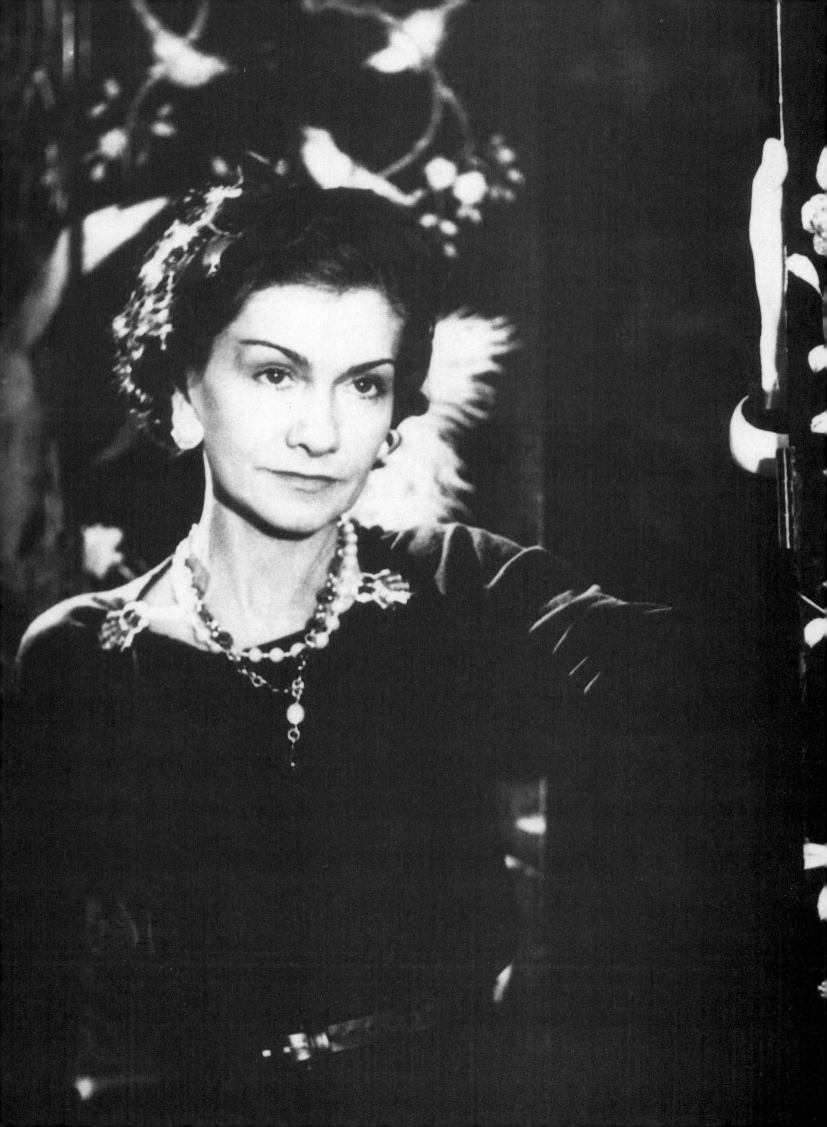

Rhinestones and Bakelite

Once upon a time . . . That's how the prettiest fairy tales begin and how the loveliest meeting in the history of costume jewelry begins, too. They met in the twenties — Bakelite and rhinestones. The avant-garde synthetic that expanded the limits of design and the stone with its penchant for opulence — it was a match made in heaven. And clever artists have done everything to

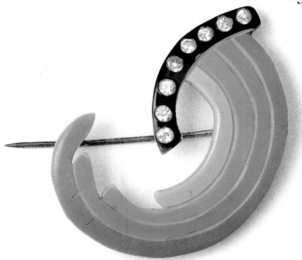

give this unique dialogue of opposites a becoming frame. Bakelite's material wealth and the rhinestone's sparkle mutually accentuate and enhance each other and allow the most fantastic images to be created: fluttering ribbons, heavy bangles, refined brooches — rhinestones lend subtle, radiant accents to Bakelite's deep colors, and provide the most exciting contrast to its clear shapes. Motifs from exotic cultures are intentionally invoked: charming Bakelite Indian brooches, pins inspired by the East. And Bakelite shines not only in pitch-black. Its turquoise, yellow, and translucent variations bring a newfound radiance to rhinestones in jewelry whose allure remains irresistible today.

R*ainbow pin, multicolored Bakelite set with rhinestones, 1935*

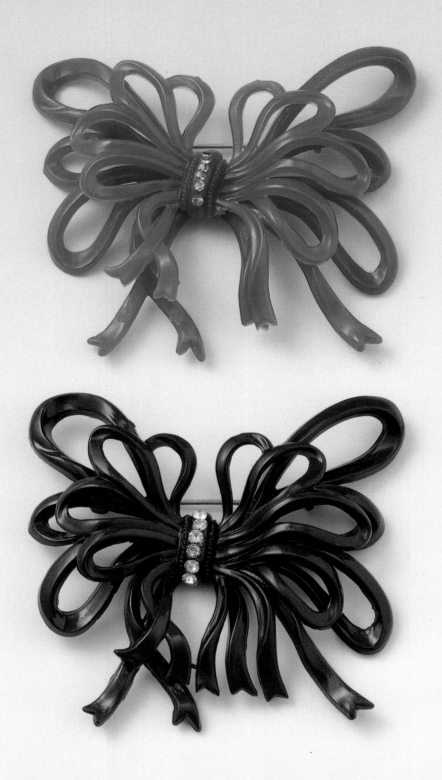

*Bakelite bow pins set with rhinestones,
both 1935*

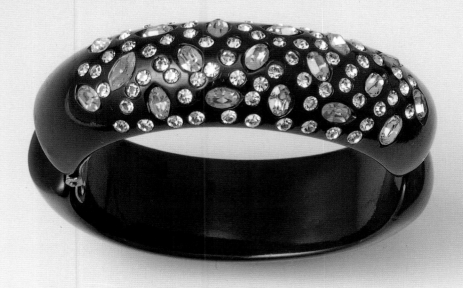

*Bakelite bangle set with
rhinestones, 1950*

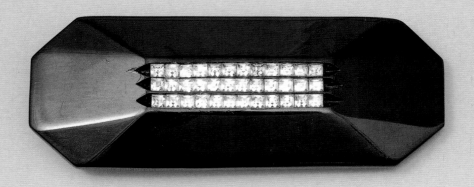

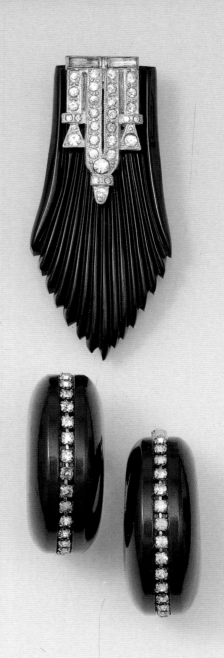

*Art Deco jewelry, black Bakelite set
with rhinestones
TOP: brooch, 1935
CENTER: brooch, 1930
BOTTOM: clip-on earrings, 1930*

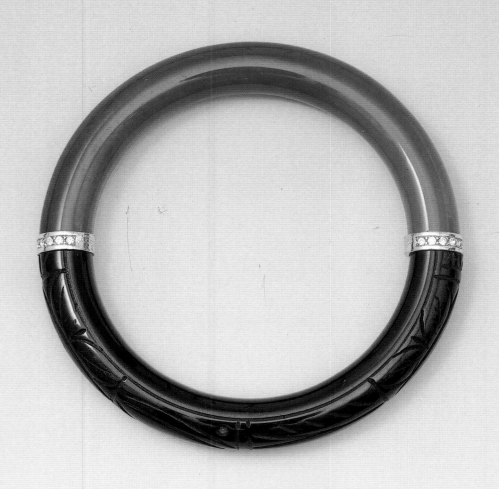

Bangle, black and red cut plastic,
signed Givenchy, *1960*

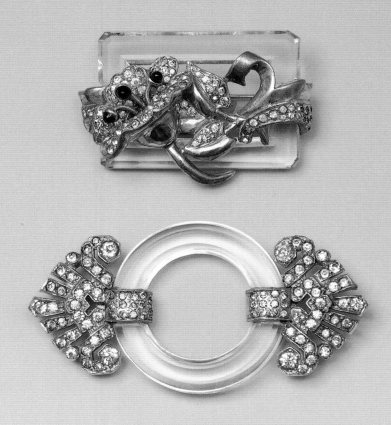

*Brooches with floral motifs, rhinestones
on lead crystal, top brooch colored gold,
both around 1935*

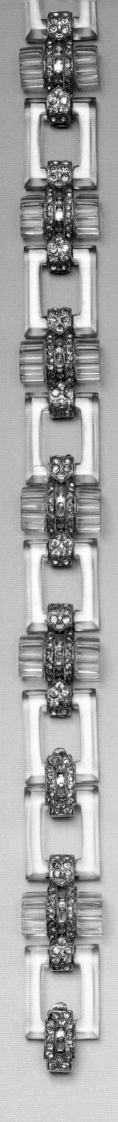

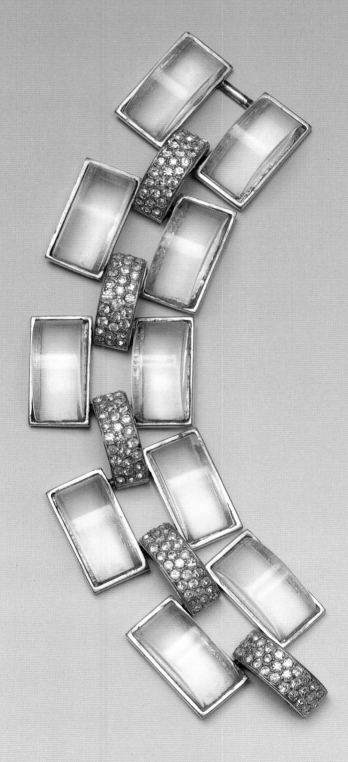

Left: necklace, rhinestones with plastic, which has turned green over time, 1930
Right: bracelet by Kenneth Jay Lane, rhinestones with acrylic, 1960

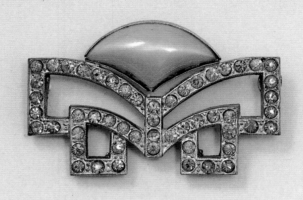

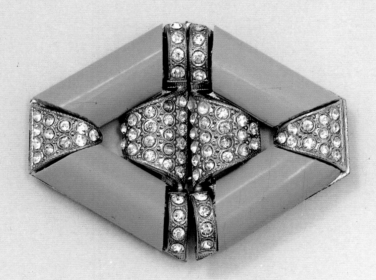

*T*OP: *Art Deco pin, rhinestones with
yellow Bakelite, 1930*
*B*OTTOM: *Art Deco belt buckle,
rhinestones with turquoise Bakelite, 1935*

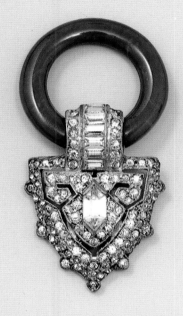

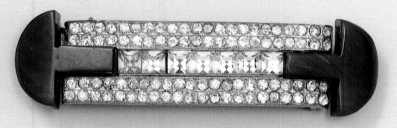

*T*OP: *Art Deco clip, green Bakelite and rhinestones, some baguette-cut, 1930*
BOTTOM: *Art Deco brooch, baguette-cut rhinestones with green Bakelite, 1930*

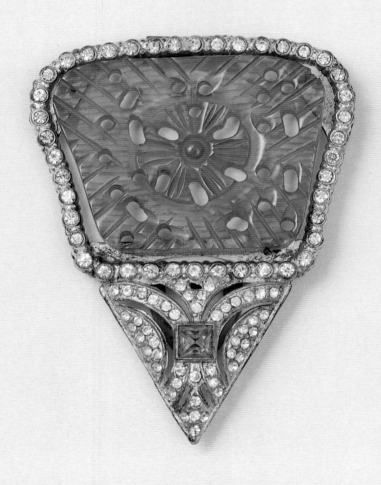

*Art Deco clip, rhinestones with topaz-
colored cut plastic, 1935*

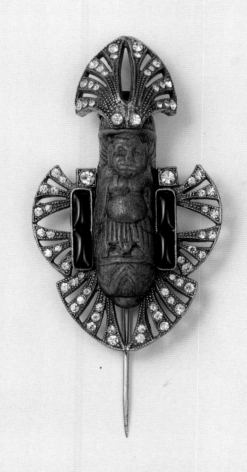

*Art Deco turban pin in Aztec-influenced
motif, rhinestones with dark green
plastic, 1928*

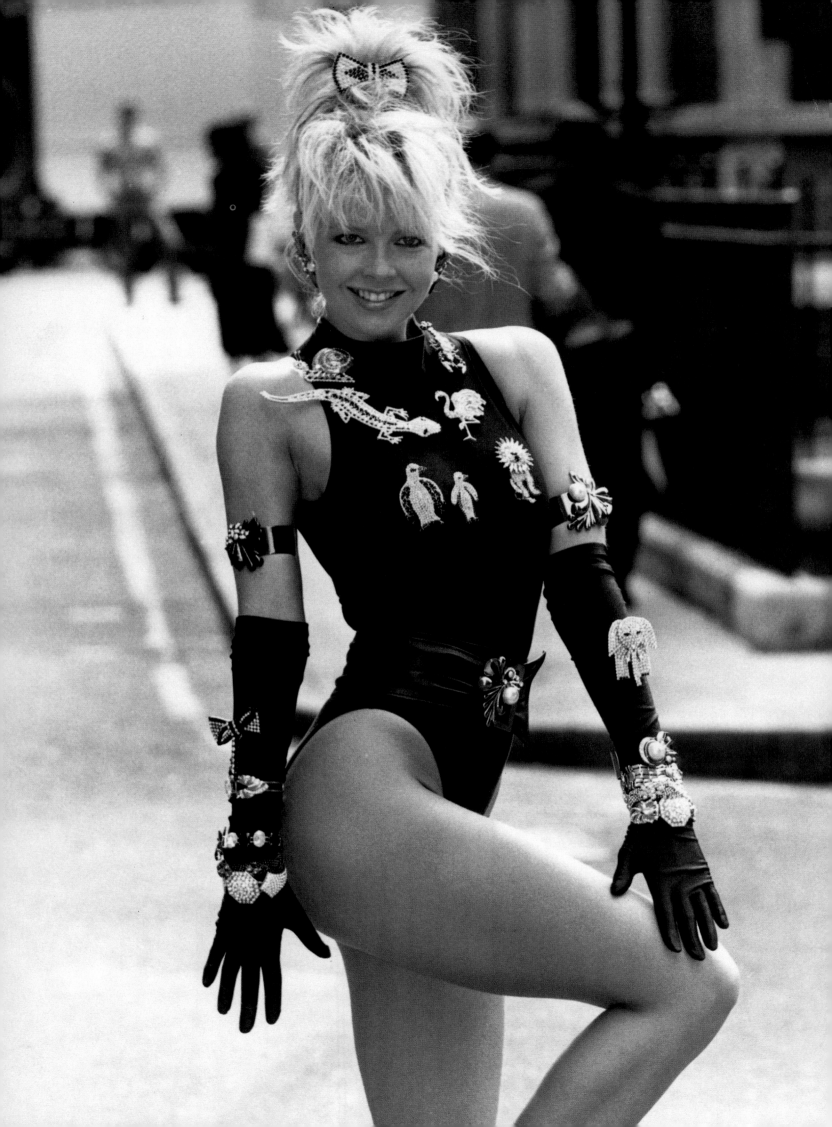

Birds

*T*heir feathers bring color to the sky, their flight induces dreams. Made of gold-colored silver or white metal and set with sparkling stones, they brighten and enliven the day. Covered in rhinestones, the prettiest brooches, clips, and earrings make for a marriage of birds: long-legged flamingos, proud peacocks, and fluttering hummingbirds rival elegant swallows and round-eyed owls. Even the tiny sparrow has a place in this colorful flock.

Rhinestone flamingo with raised wings, pin, 1935

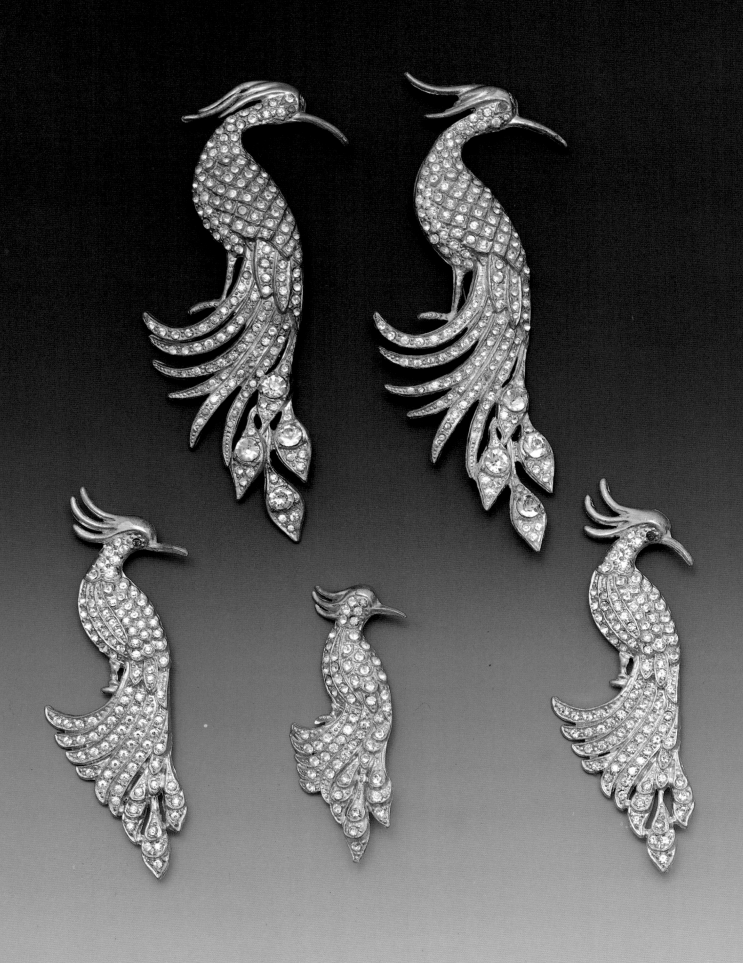

*Five very similar bird-of-paradise pins,
white rhinestones on metal, all 1935*

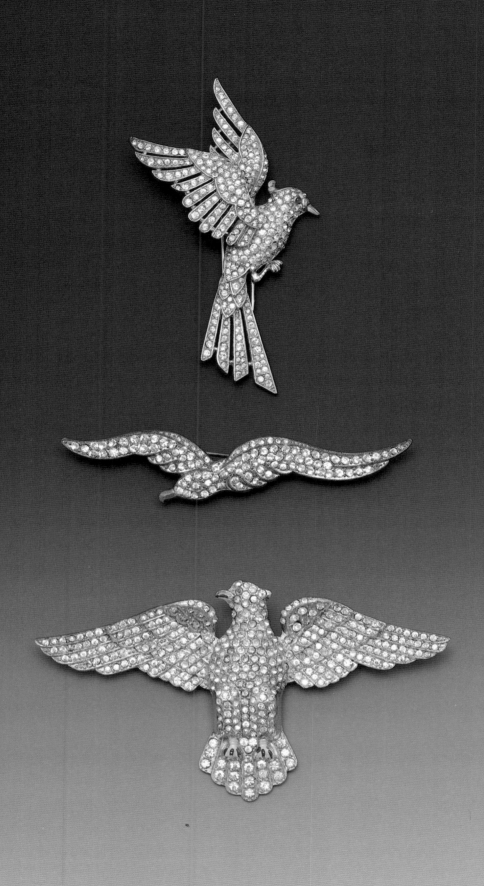

*T*OP: *landing jay, signed* Trifari, *1940*
CENTER: *Sea gull pin, white*
rhinestones, 1930
BOTTOM: *American bald eagle pin, 1940*

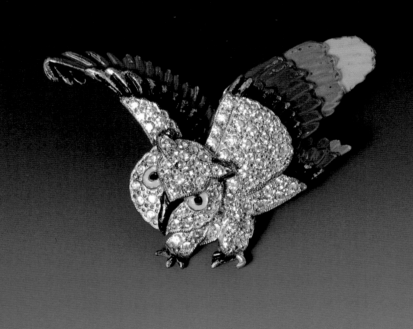

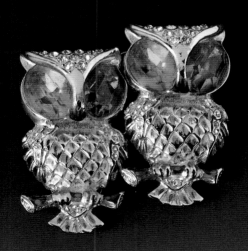

OPPOSITE: owl on the prowl, white
rhinestones with painted metal,
brooch, 1952
ABOVE: owl clip-on earrings, signed
Coro Duette, *1950*

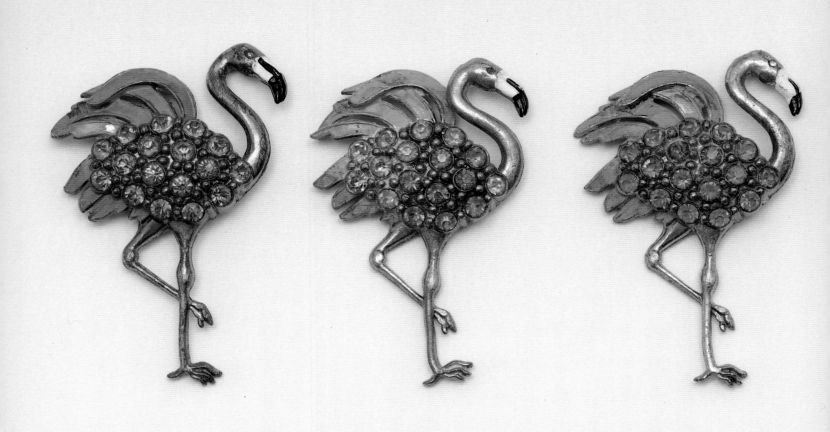

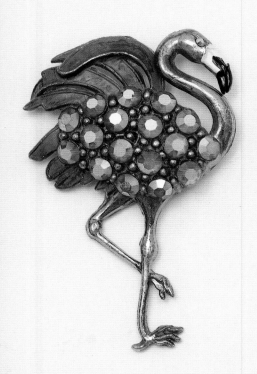
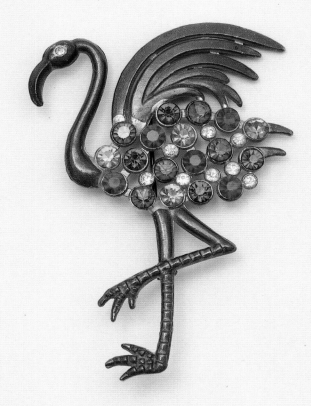

*Flamingo pins set with colored
rhinestones on painted metal, all 1940*

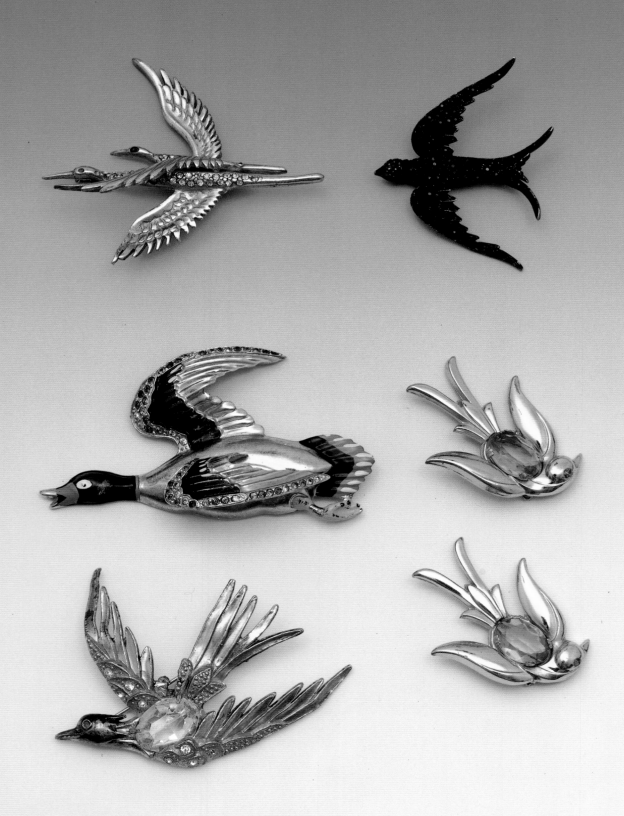

Bird pins, 1940–45
CENTER AND BOTTOM, RIGHT: *two
striking swallows, rhinestones and light
blue glass set in gold-colored sterling
silver, signed* Coro, *1940*

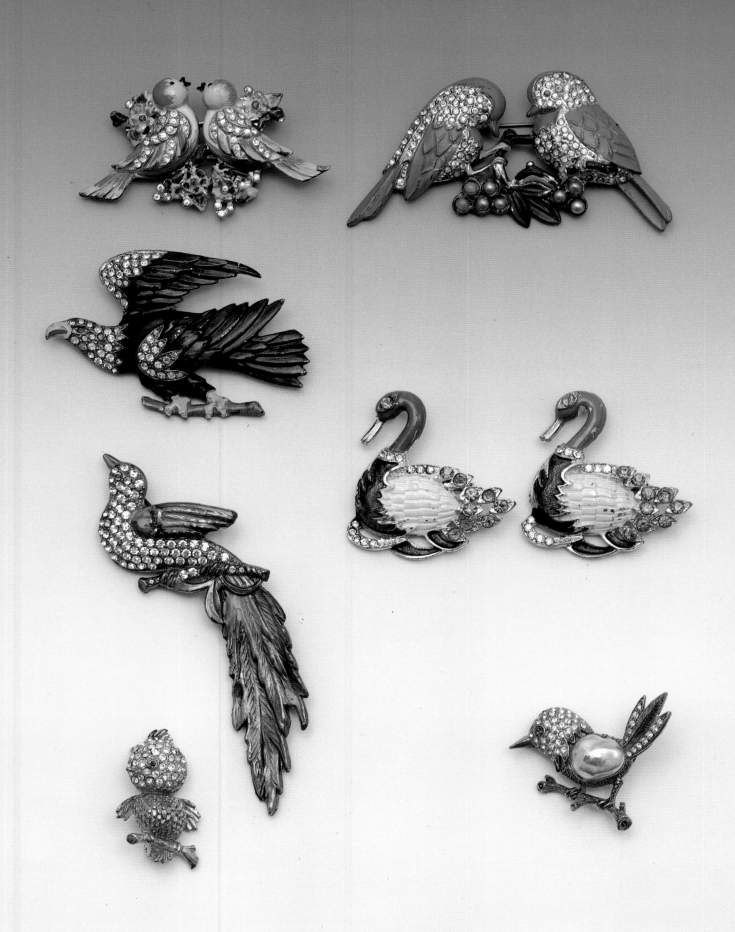

*Various bird pins, all 1935–40;
the two ducks, center right, can be
connected with a brass link*

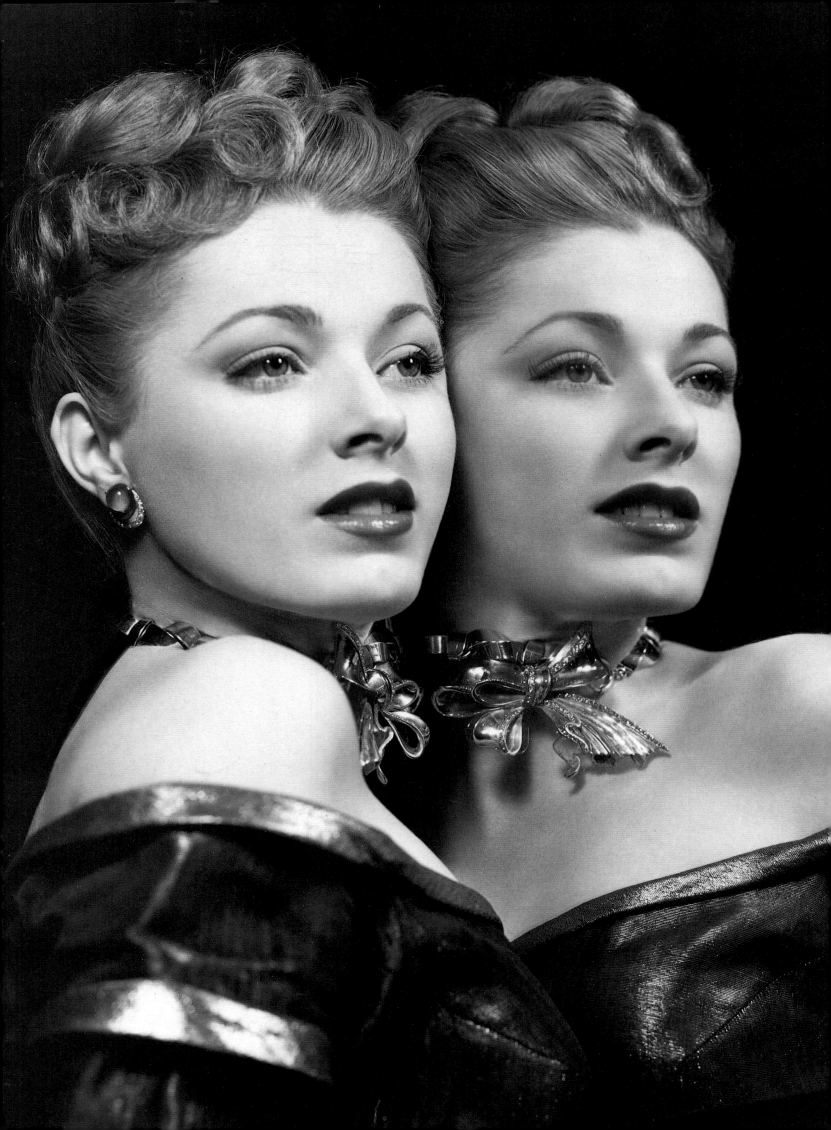

Bows

At one time a wardrobe was unthinkable without them. Large or small, stiff or silky and flowing, they are the epitome of feminine elegance. Casual fashion dispensed with the fabric bow as an accessory long ago — and wondrously

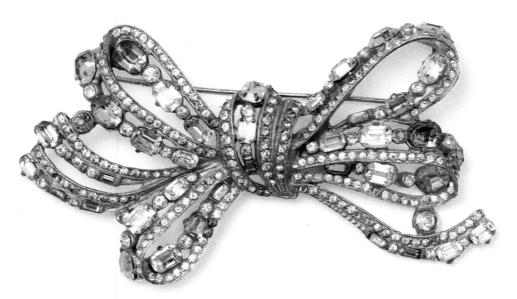

rediscovered it as a rhinestone-covered, entwined gold ribbon. Lavishly decorated, it gives a slightly ironic undertone to the play of possibilities.

Extravagant bow pin, white rhinestones, 1940

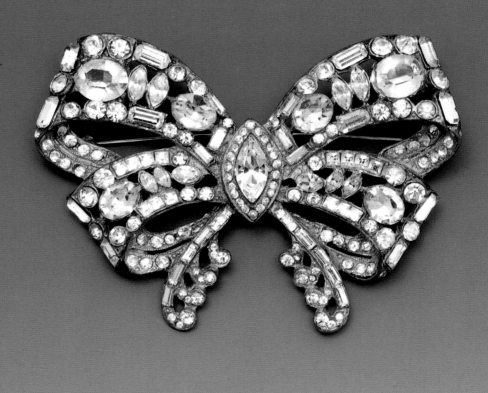

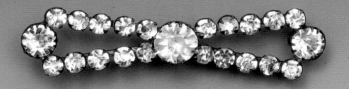

*T*OP: *large symmetrical bow pin, 1940*
*B*OTTOM: *bow pin, rhinestones, 1910*

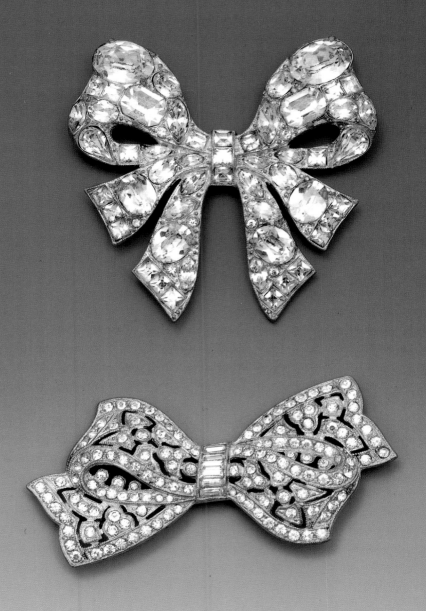

*T*OP: *decorative rhinestone bow pin, 1935*
*B*OTTOM: *rhinestone bow pin, 1935*

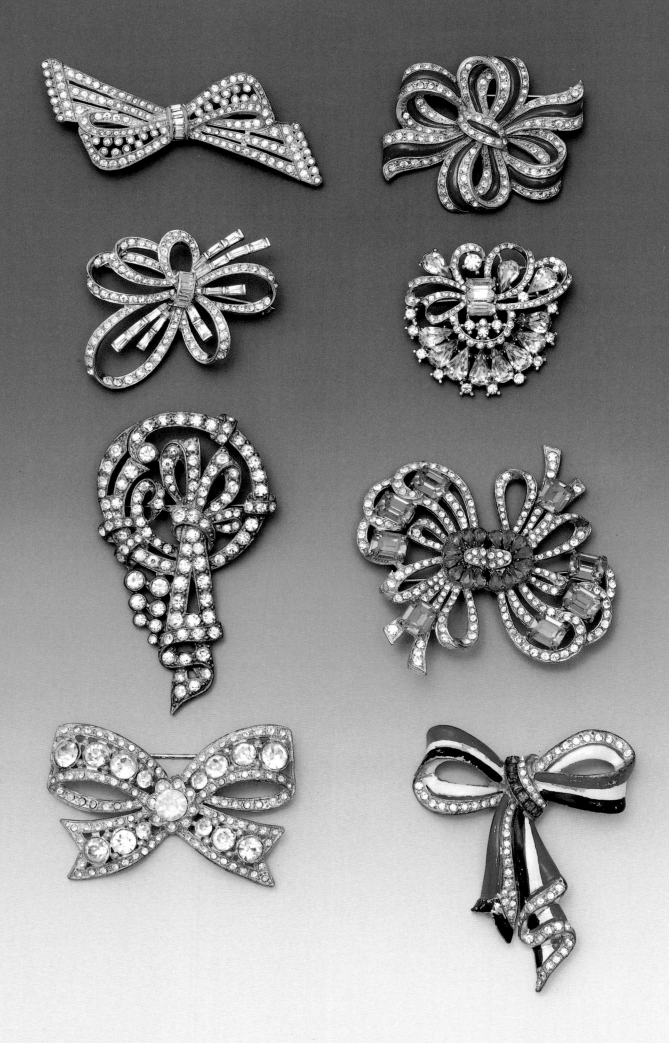

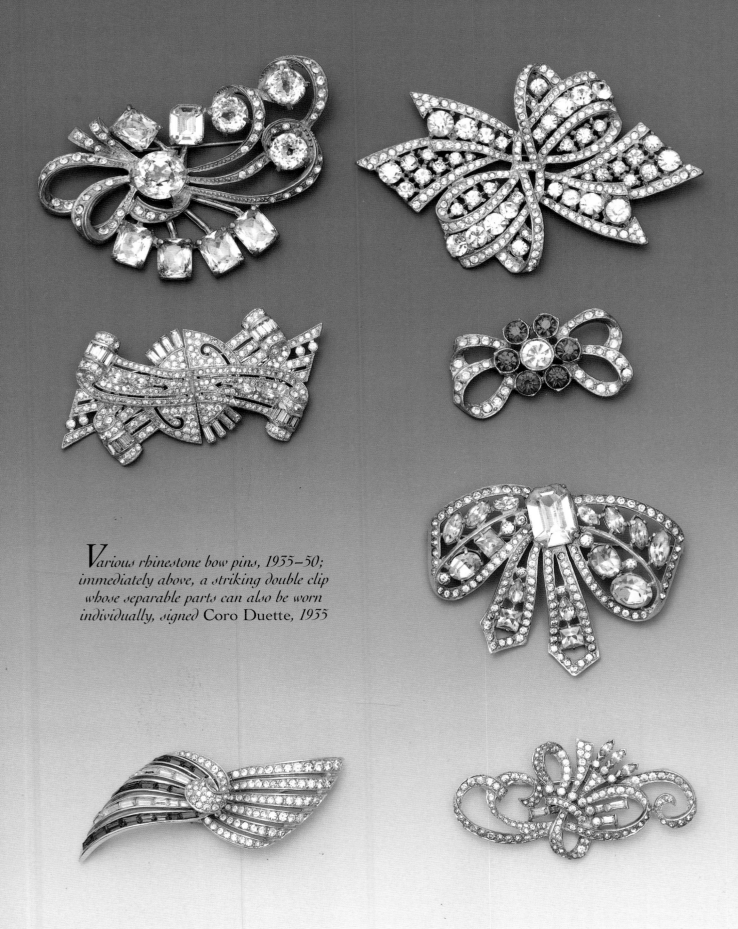

Various rhinestone bow pins, 1935–50; immediately above, a striking double clip whose separable parts can also be worn individually, signed Coro Duette, 1935

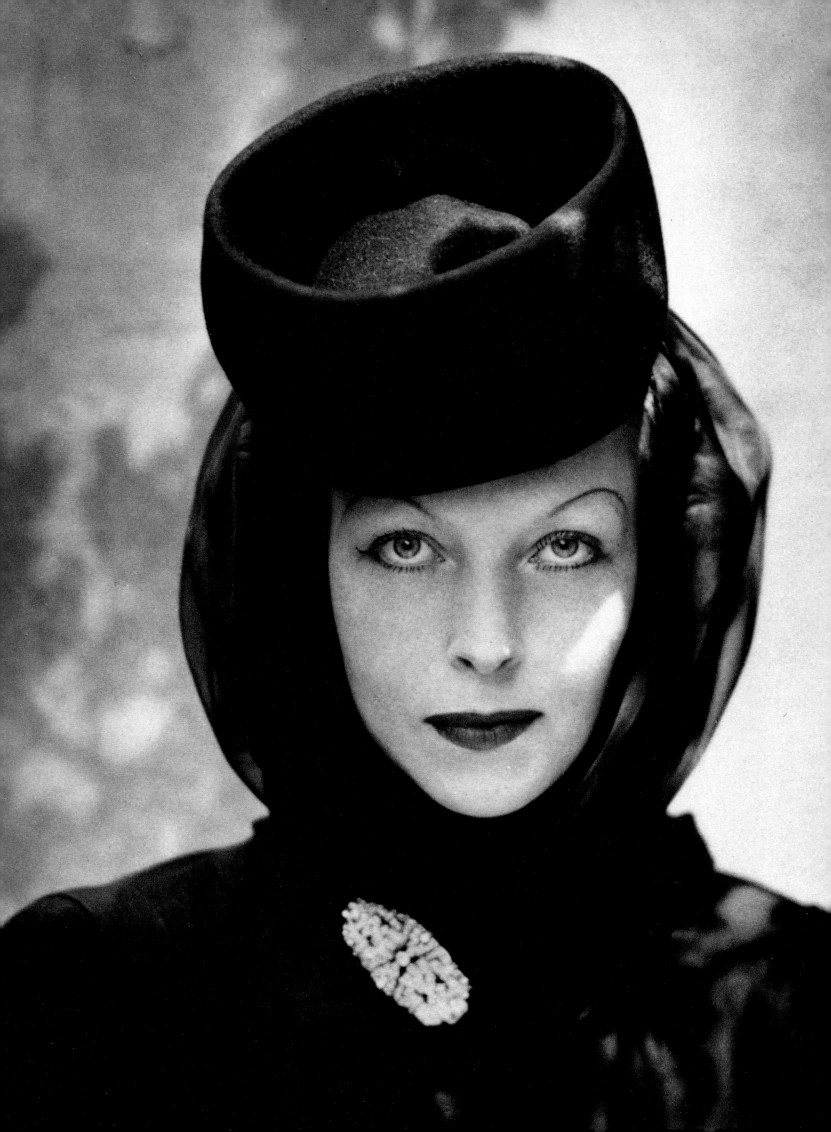

Feathers

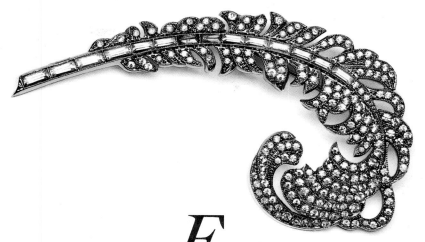

*E*legant homage to a thing of beauty. Illusively weightless and ready to blow away, strikingly simulated in metal and glass. Rhinestones and the art of the goldsmith make it possible. Filigree creations that inspire an impetuous desire to decorate oneself freely with outlandish feathers. The heron's feather in miniature — certainly it serves courtship well. Not only in the country but in our modern metropolitan jungles, too, the feather clearly symbolizes the successful hunt.

Feather pin, white rhinestones, 1935

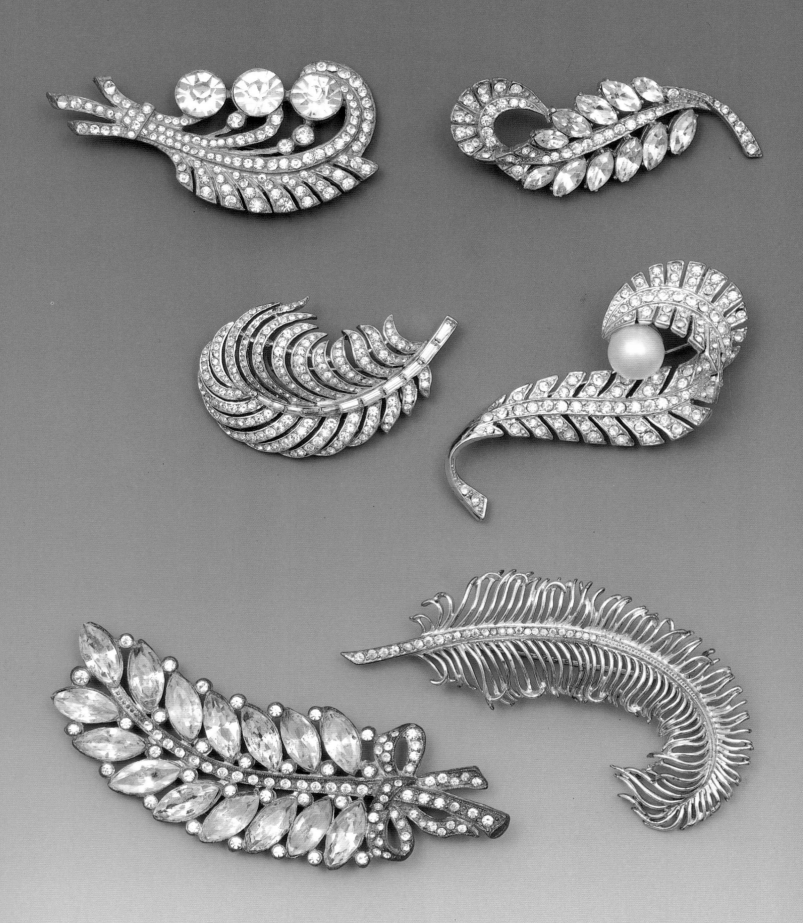

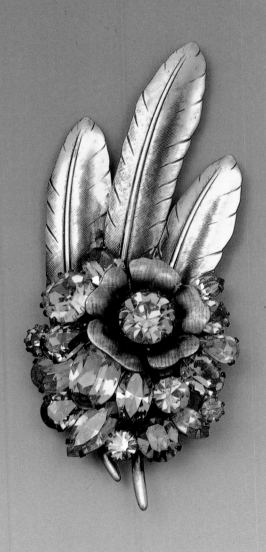

*OPPOSITE: various rhinestone feather
pins, all 1935–40
ABOVE: feather brooch, topaz-colored
rhinestones on brass, signed
Vendôme, 1945*

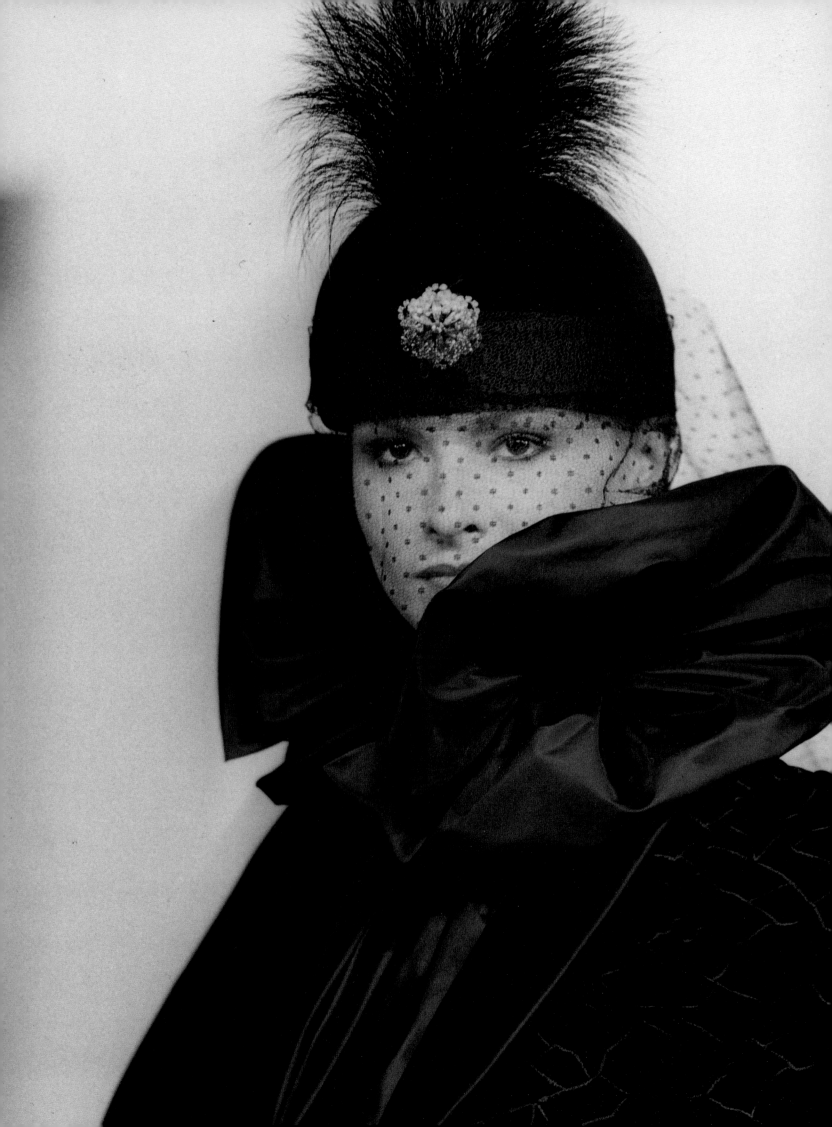

Flower Baskets

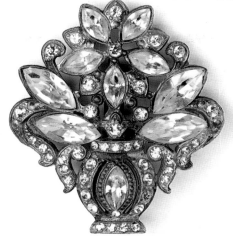

*I*n the good old days chivalrous gentlemen sent their sweethearts the most beautiful flowers in baskets. Rhinestones recapture this charming gesture, giving it a touch of timelessness. Elegantly woven of metal ribbons or cut in twinkling crystal, these dainty baskets can hardly hold their bountiful bouquets. Abundantly filled cornucopias in the Renaissance style bring back memories of sumptuous festivals under radiant skies. To imitate nature and yet to stylize it — herein lies the magic of this jewelry.

*F*lower basket brooch, rhinestones, 1938

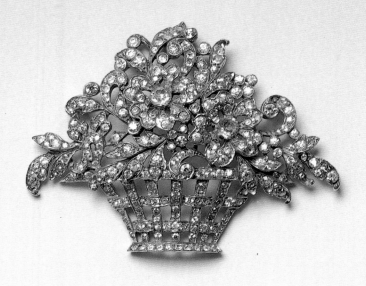

*ABOVE: flower basket, white rhinestones
on gold-colored white metal, signed
Trifari, 1940
OPPOSITE: flower basket brooches,
1930–35*

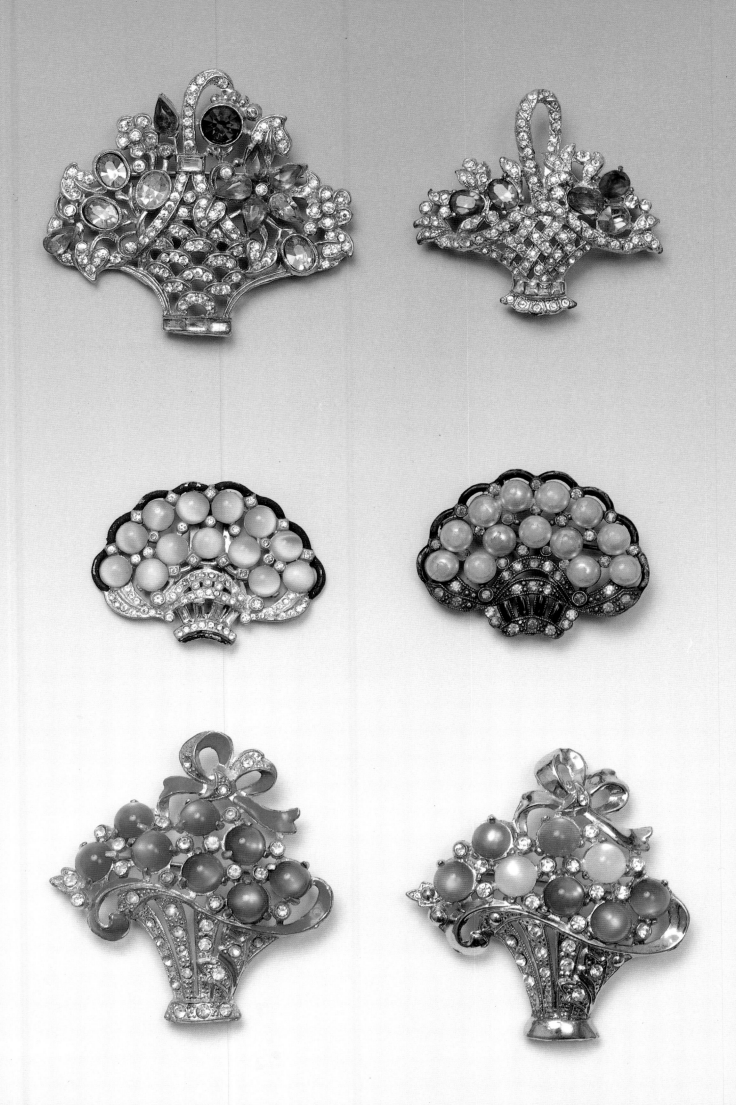

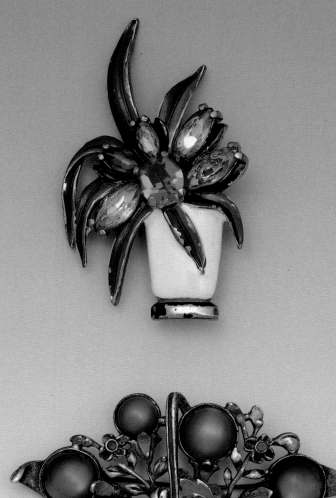

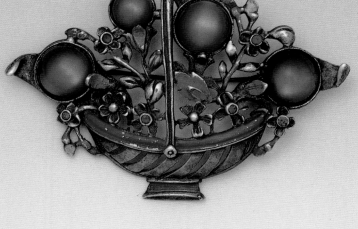

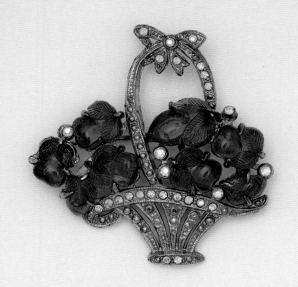

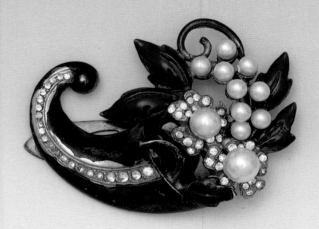

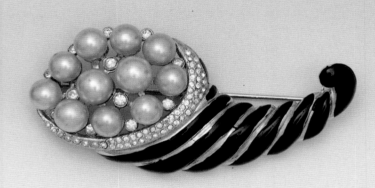

*Opposite, top: an agave, rhinestones
with painted metal, 1940
Center: flower basket, 1930
Bottom: flower basket, signed
Coro, 1930
Above: cornucopia brooches, rhinestones
and imitation pearls on colored metal
Left: 1930
Right: 1940*

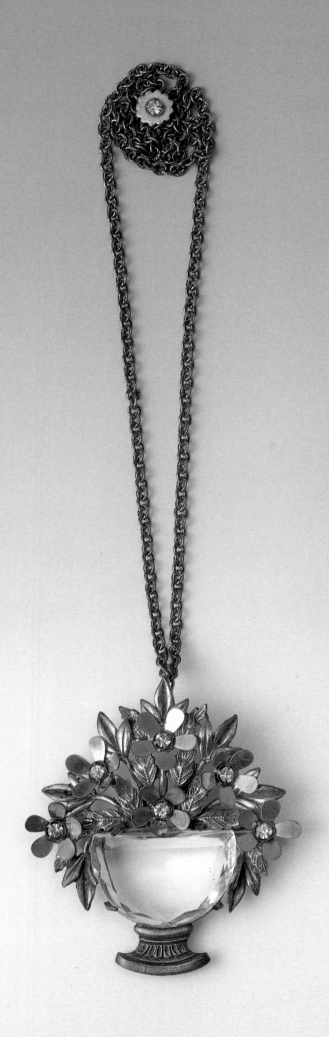

Rhinestone flower basket necklace, 1900

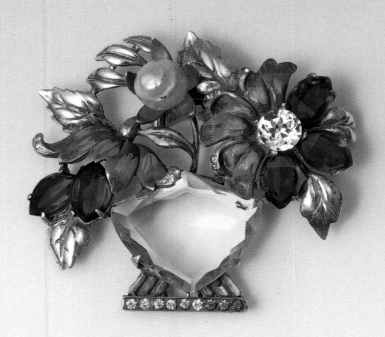

*Flower basket brooch, rhinestones with
acrylic, 1940*

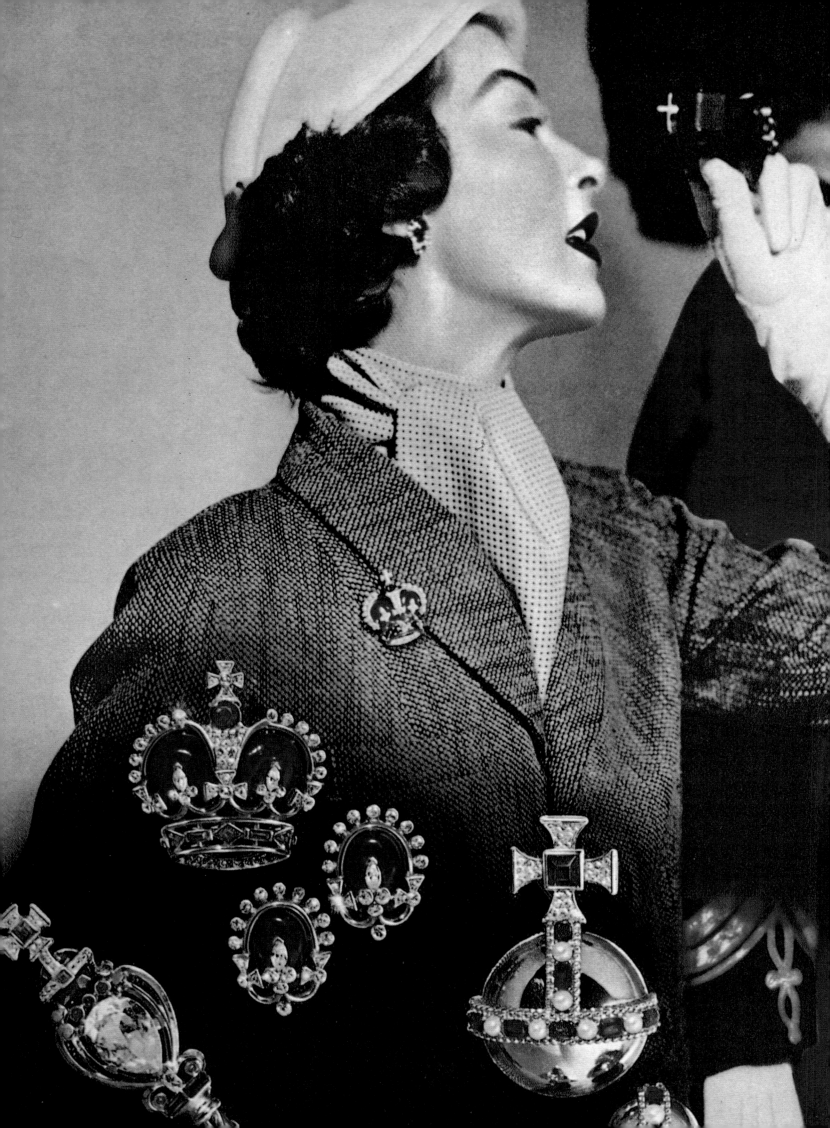

National Emblems

The philosophy of rhinestones taken to an extreme — thanks to the rhinestone, diamonds are within the reach of everyone, not only the wealthy and powerful, who once so lavishly ornamented themselves. Long-revered and sacrosanct, insignia of power are now boldly replicated in our democratic century. Royal crowns, swords, flags, even clerical symbols adorn casual shirts and most of all bare skin. And why not, when in the meanwhile the motto has become: What price the world?

Sword, white rhinestones on metal, 1920

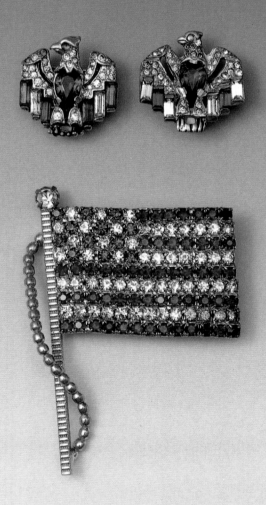

TOP: *American bald eagle pins*
BOTTOM: *Old Glory brooch, 1935*

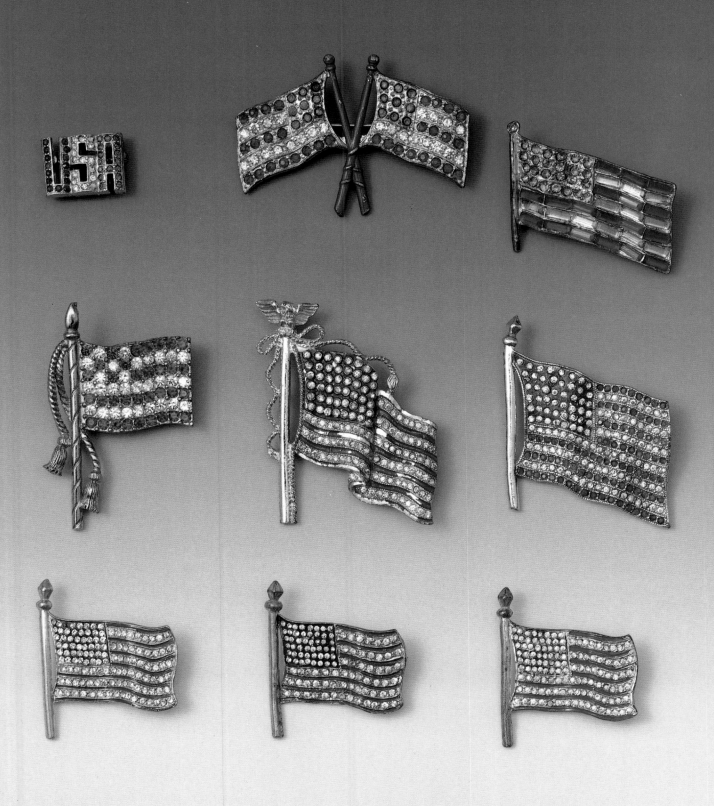

USA pin, double flag, and various Old Glory flags, 1935–40; of particular interest: Old Glory, top right, rhinestones and baguette-cut rhinestones, 1920

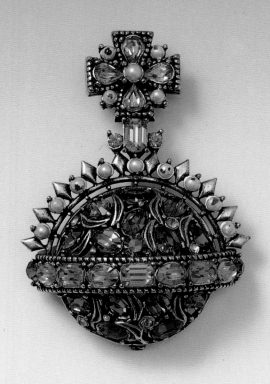

*Imperial orb, rhinestones with imitation
pearls on gold-colored metal, 1950*

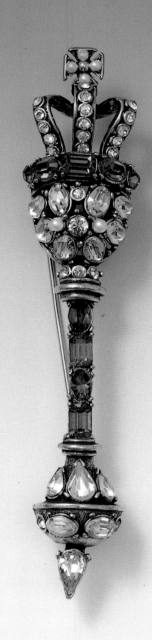

*S*cepter pin, violet rhinestones on
metal, 1950

*Various crown pins, white rhinestones
with colored cabochons, 1940–60*

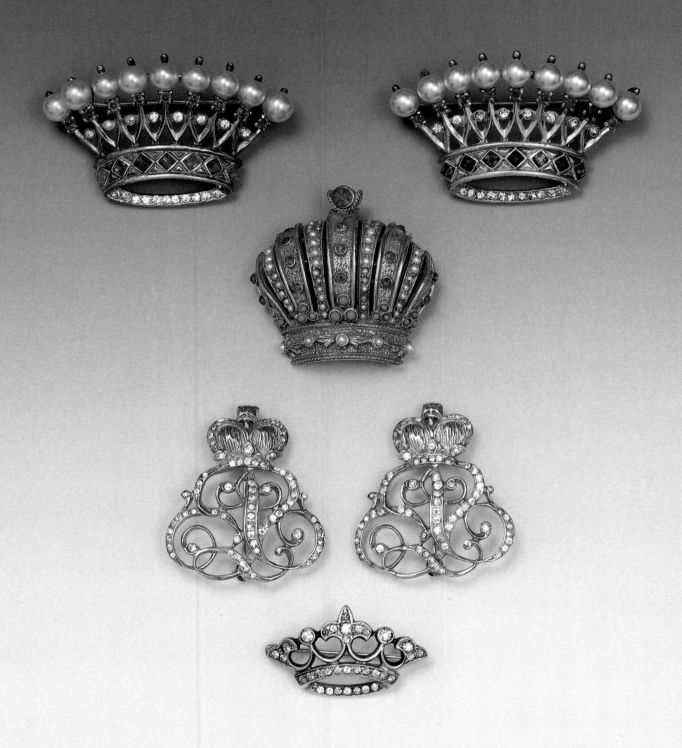

*T*OP: *crowns of rhinestones and
imitation pearls on gold-colored silver, 1945*
CENTER: *Russian crown, 1960*
SECOND ROW FROM BOTTOM: *Big
Cotton Carnival Society symbol,
rhinestones on gold-colored silver,
engraved 1948*
BOTTOM: *small crown, rhinestones on
white metal, 1950*

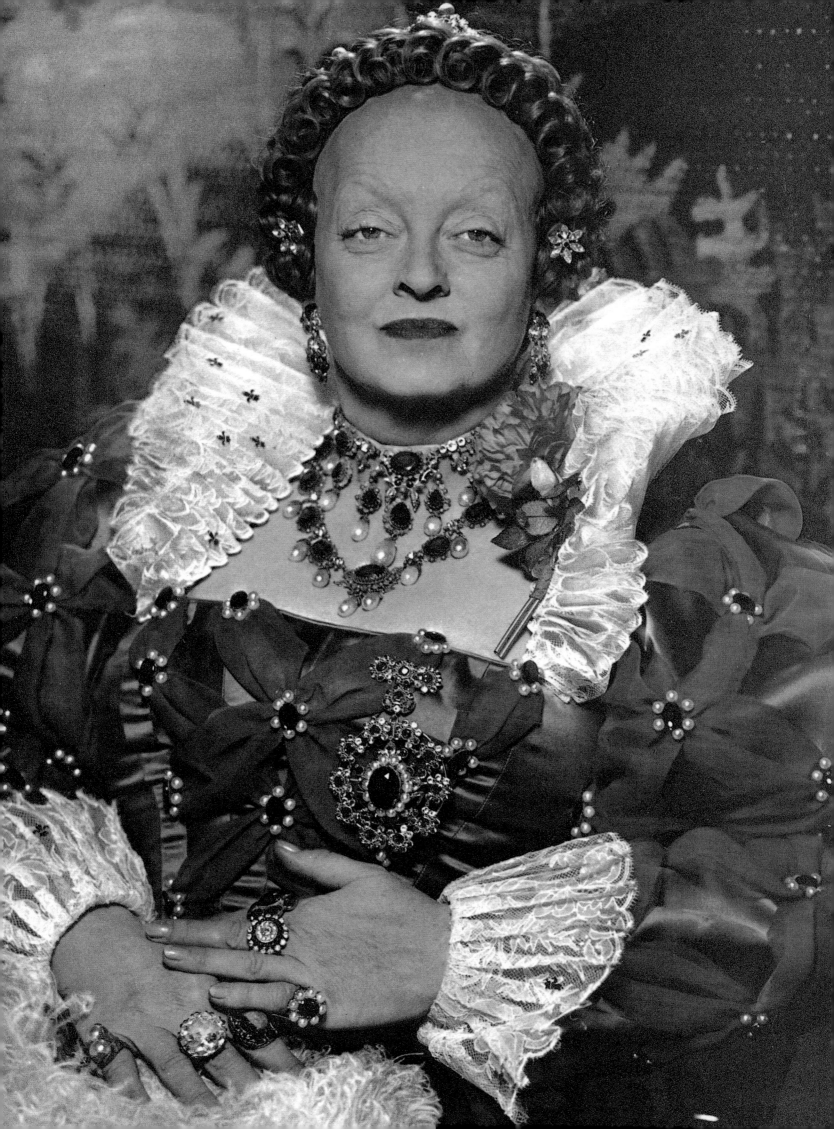

Victorian Brooches

Around the turn of the century all of Europe lived in a prim bourgeois manner, all the while yearning for the enchanting magnificence of the Orient and its sensual luxuries. Extravagant brooches revealed secret desires, reminiscent of old Constantinople and Cairo, of the legendary goldsmiths of the bazaars. With their intricately artful forms, their large shimmering, seductive stones of all colors, they seem lifted directly from the treasure chests of *A Thousand and One Nights,* irresistible invitations to coquettish costuming.

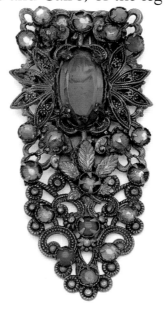

Clothing clip, colored rhinestones set in brass, 1900

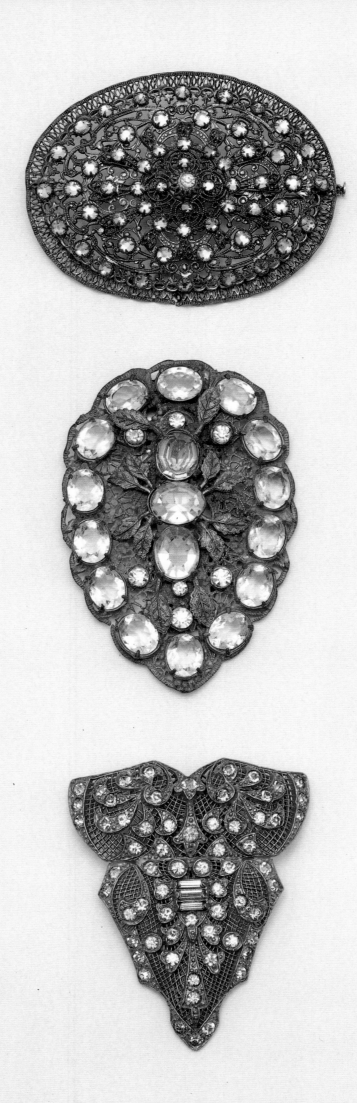

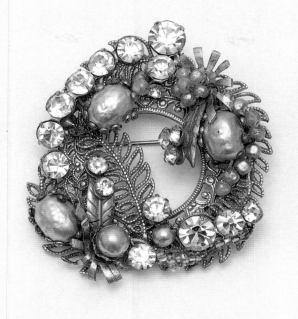

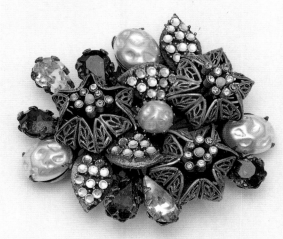

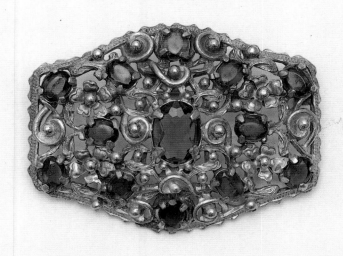

*Victorian rhinestone brooches set in brass
filigree, all 1900–1910*

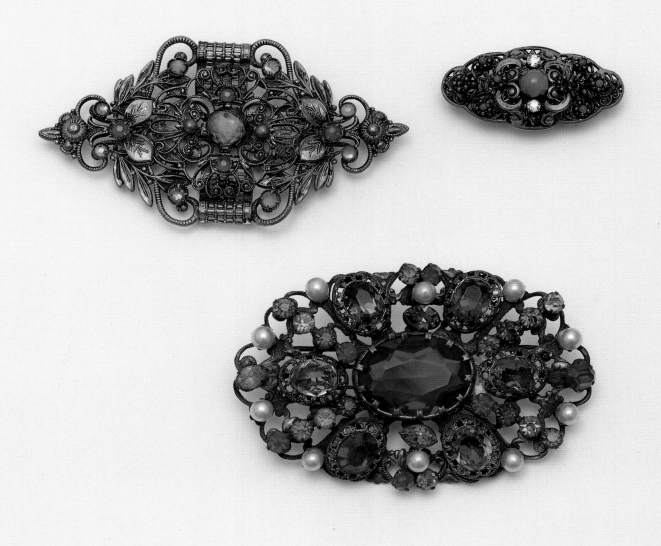

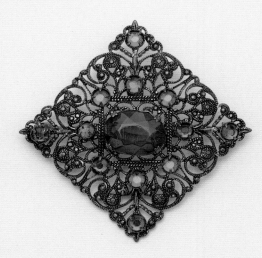

*F*ine filigree rhinestone brooches in
historically inspired styles, created
1900–1905, with the exception of the
brooch opposite, top left, 1930

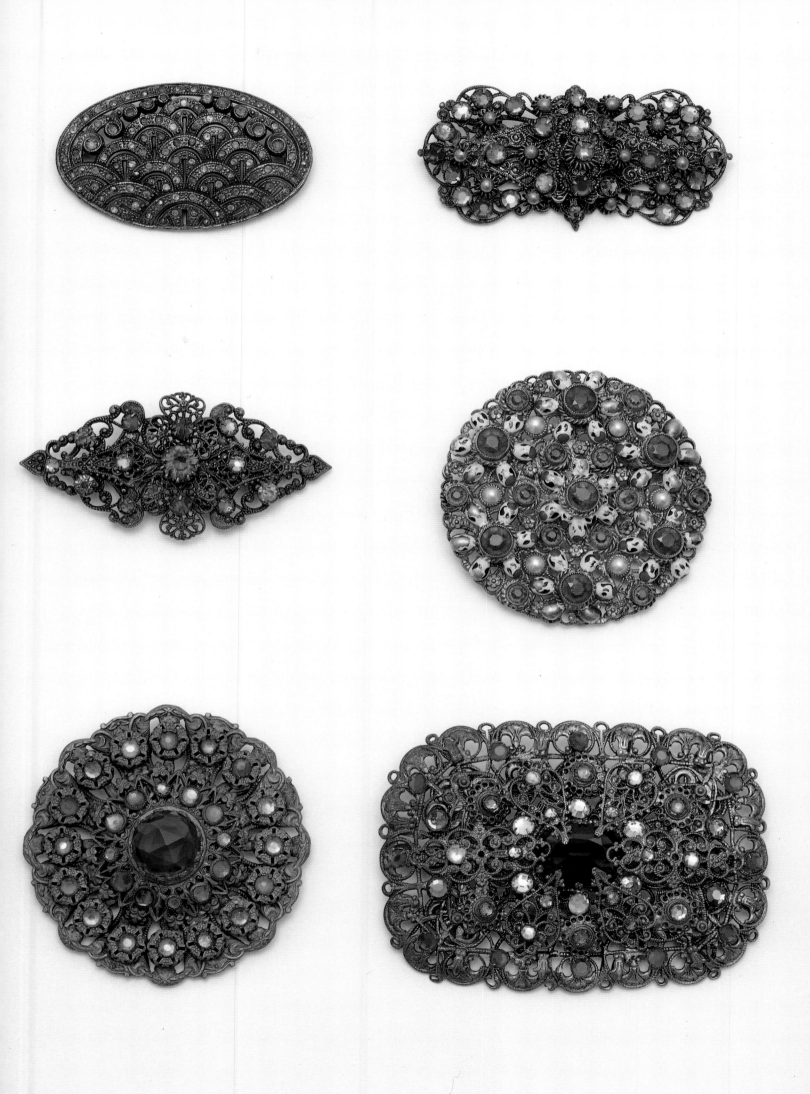

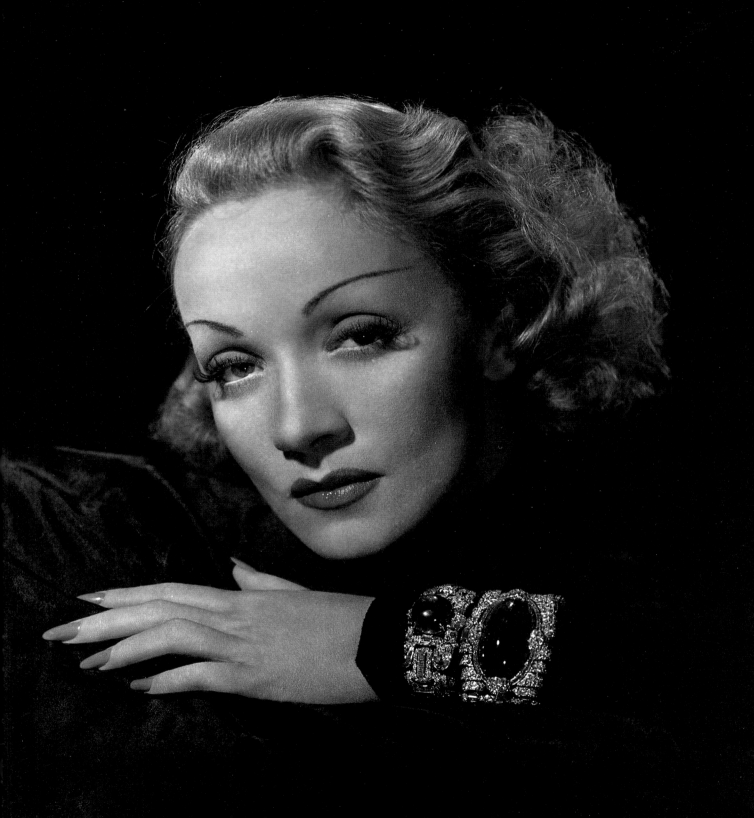

Art Deco Brooches

*I*n 1930 art and craft achieved a unique high point: aesthetics and function, long separated, melded in a breathtaking symbiosis. Jewelry designers borrowed avant-garde concepts from Erté and Le Corbusier. The clear,

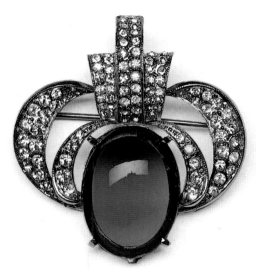

strong forms of their pieces anticipated the ideal woman, who now came into being: a woman conscious of her jewelry and clothing, yet in control of her life. For the first time artificial materials were deliberately set, and rhinestones celebrated a new heyday. Frequently only a few stones with enormous refraction were used, in classical combinations with horn and plastic, in arrow-shaped brooches. No wonder this stylish jewelry is in vogue once again.

*M*odern brooch in the Art Deco
style, 1960

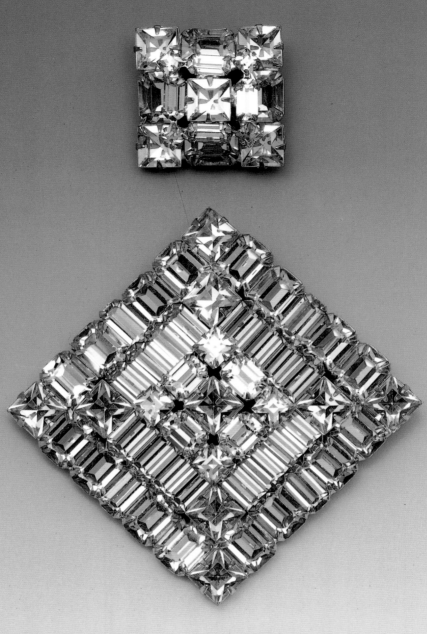
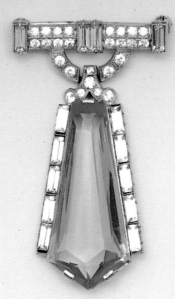

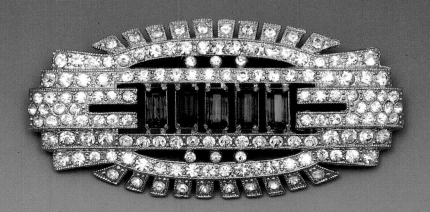

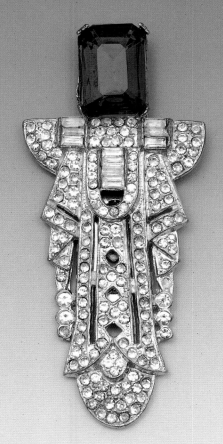

*O*PPOSITE, TOP AND CENTER: *brooches
of light blue baguette-cut rhinestones,
1940–55*
BOTTOM: *exquisite brooch with drop-
shaped pendant, 1935*
ABOVE, TOP: *Art Deco brooch, signed
Coro, 1935*
BOTTOM: *rhinestone clip with dark blue
keystone, 1935*

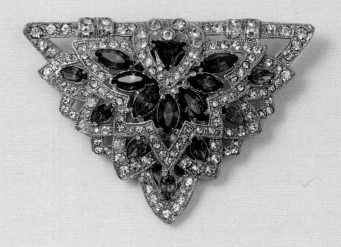

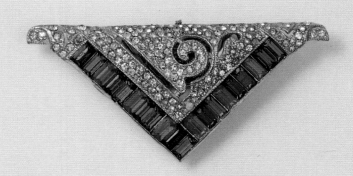

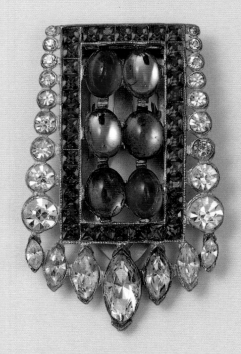

*T*OP: *Art Deco brooch, 1935*
CENTER: *classic Art Deco brooch, 1935*
BOTTOM: *Art Deco brooch, rhinestones*
with multicolored cabochons, 1935

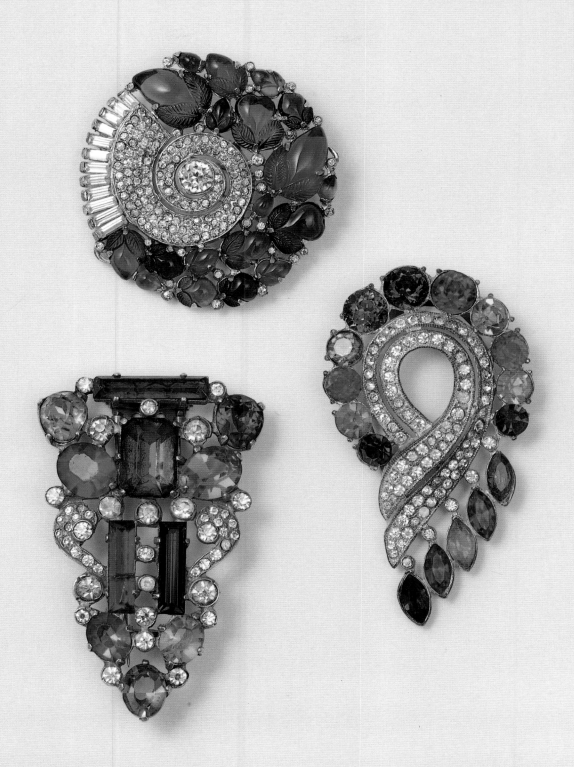

*T*op: *unsigned designer piece,*
rhinestones with colored cut glass, 1940
*R*ight: *brooch in the shape of a question*
mark, 1935
*L*eft: *Art Deco clip, rhinestones set in*
sterling silver, 1940

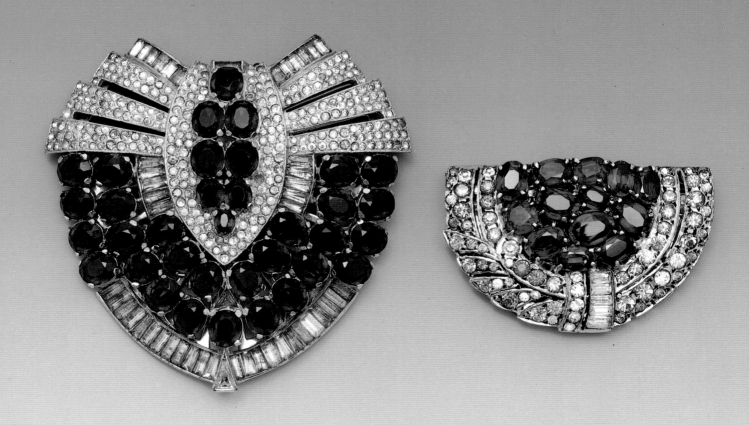

*L*EFT: *mask type rhinestone clip with
cut-glass stones, signed* TKF, *1935*
*R*IGHT: *semicircular rhinestone clip, 1935*

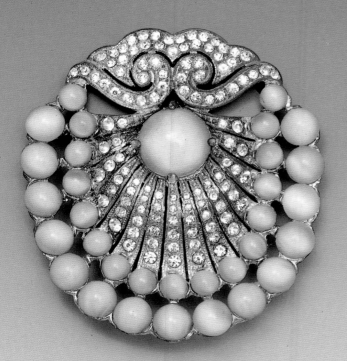
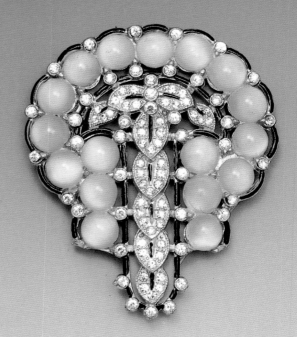

*Two Art Deco brooches with light blue
glass cabochons, both 1935*

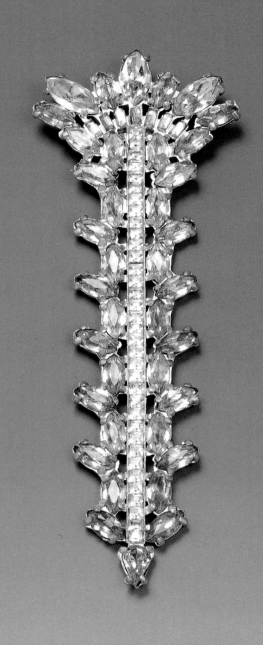

*L*arge rhinestone pin in architectural
design, signed Artex, 1935

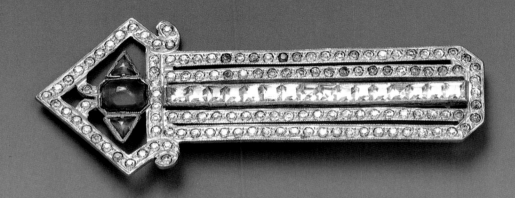

*A*rt Deco pin in architectural
design, 1930

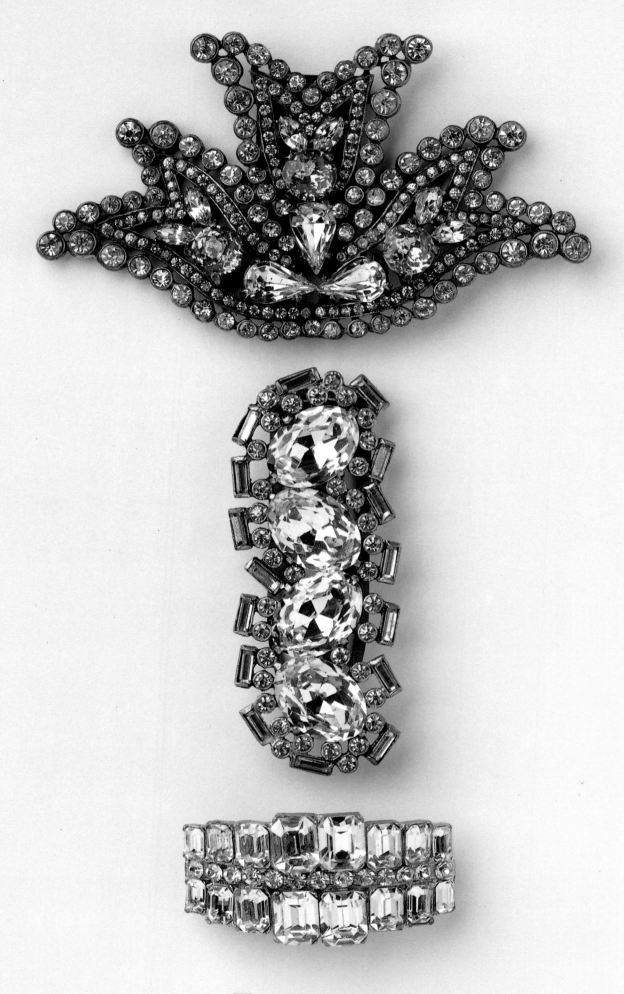

*T*OP: *rhinestone clip, 1900*
*C*ENTER: *rhinestone brooch, 1935*
*B*OTTOM: *rhinestone brooch, 1935*

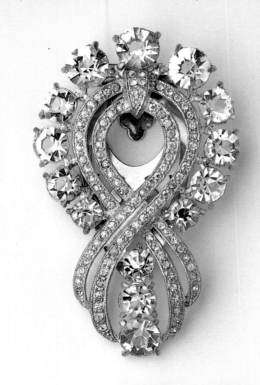

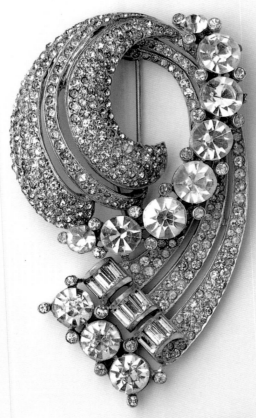

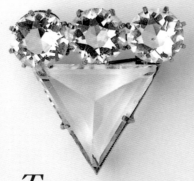

TOP: rhinestone clip, 1935
CENTER: decorative rhinestone brooch,
signed Coro, 1935
BOTTOM: brooch, 1935

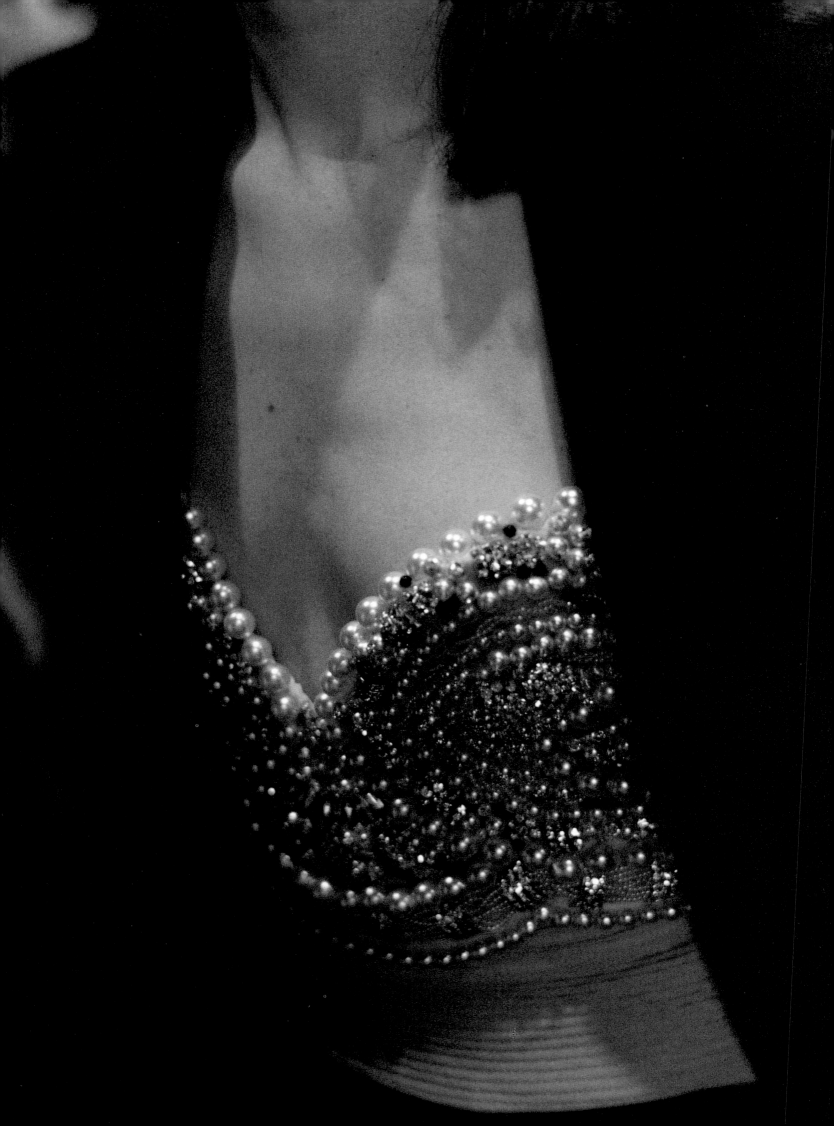

Fruit

*A*pples, cherries, grapes, colorfully lacquered and covered with rhinestones — paradisiacal showpieces pretty enough to eat. No wonder Eve managed to tempt Adam to stray from

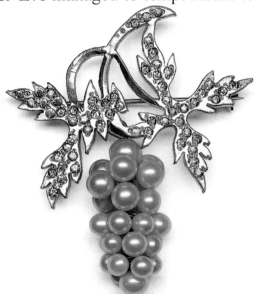

the path of virtue with a piece of fruit. Who wouldn't have weakened at the sight of such a glowing little morsel? For rhinestone enthusiasts there is a virtual Garden of Eden, inviting both indulgence and the temptation of picking a piece for oneself. A whole harvest of unusual, beguiling fruits creates an appetite for wearing them in the workaday world. And best of all: there is something for every taste — tart or sweet, deliciously fresh or ripe and juicy.

Grape pin, rhinestones and faux pearls, 1955

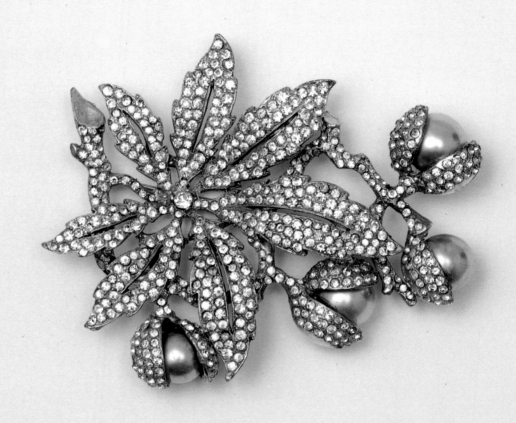

*L*eaf of white rhinestones, buds of faux
pearls, 1955

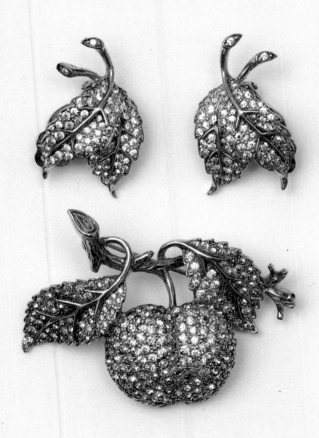

*Apple brooch with matching earrings,
white rhinestones, 1940*

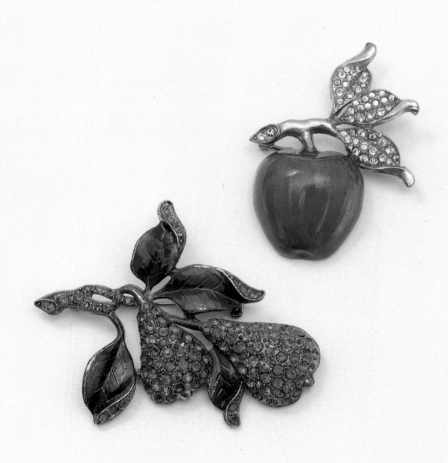

*Apple and pear pins, rhinestones and
painted metal, 1938*

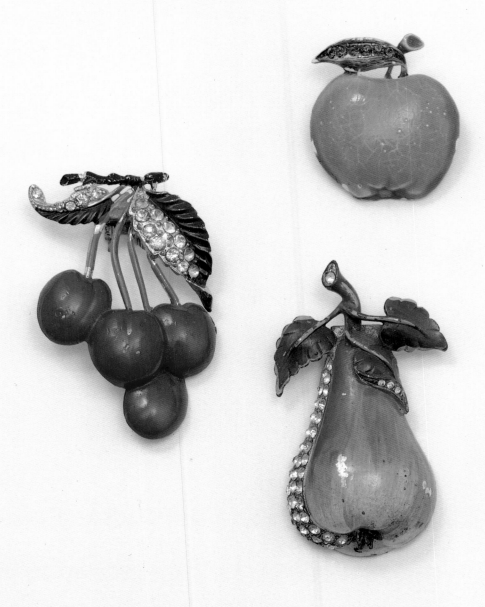

*Pin and clips, in the shape of an apple,
signed Weiss, a pear, and cherries;
rhinestones and painted metal, all 1935*

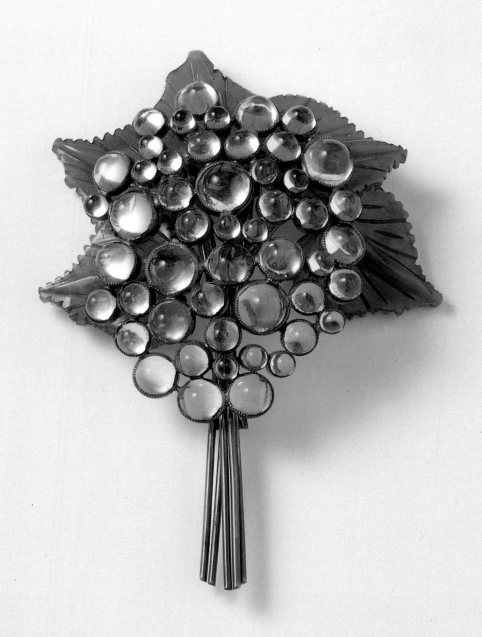

*Grape cluster, rhinestone cabochons on
metal, 1938*

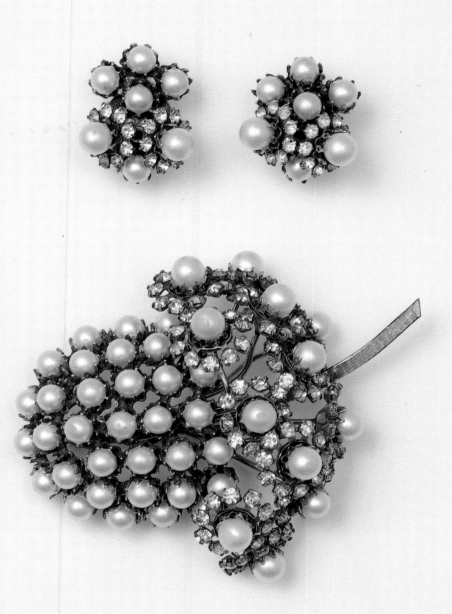

*Grape pin and matching earrings,
rhinestones and faux pearls, 1938*

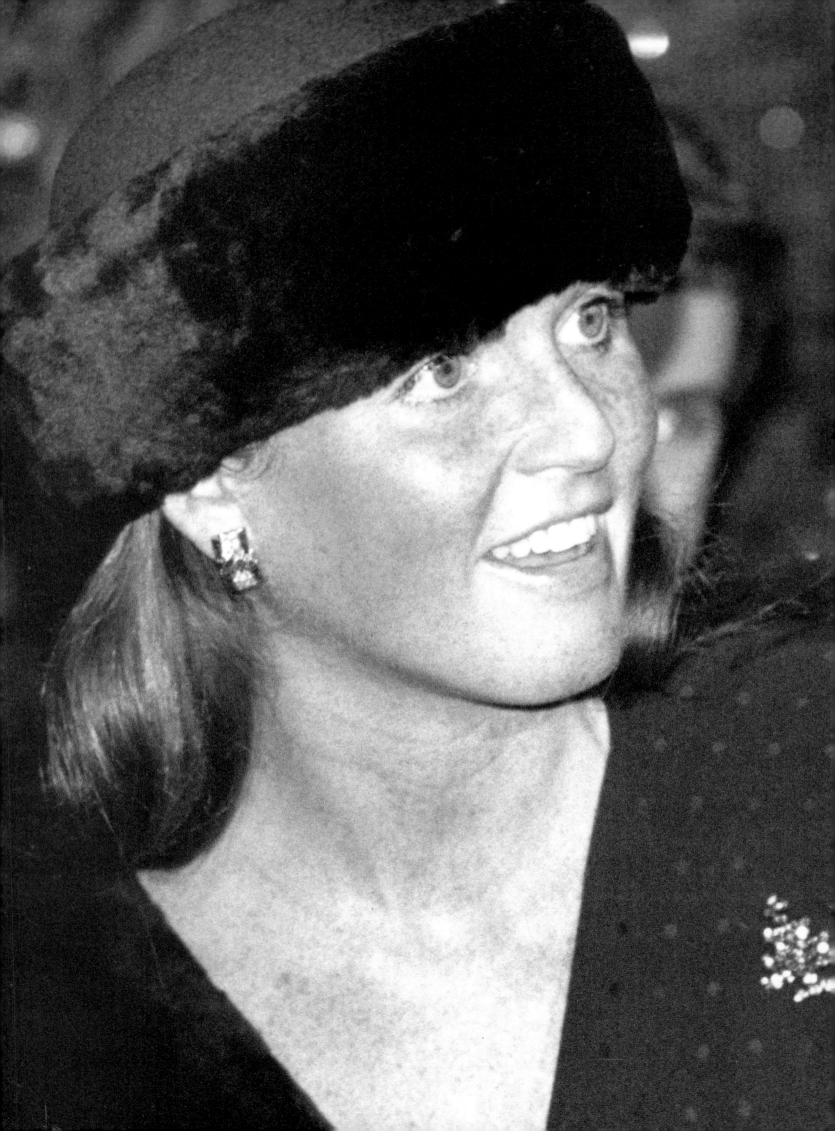

Christmas

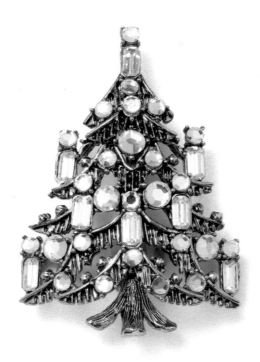

No holiday calls for jewelry more! And so miniature Christmas trees, bedecked with candles, balls, and stars twinkle and sparkle, trying to outdo their big cousins. And not just at Christmastime. They make the old childhood dream finally come true: it can be Christmas all year round. Even the Princess of York couldn't resist a shimmering spruce and wears it with as much delight as if it were the crown jewels. Inventive rhinestone designers such as Weiss and Hollycraft design a new Christmas tree every year, in everything from realistic versions to geometric interpretations. In the 1940s a small group of American collectors of everything having to do with Christmas even organized into a club: Saint Nick's shoes, Santa Claus with his jolly beard, holly wreaths made of jewels brimming with gold, and last but not least the familiar Christmas plate.

Rhinestone Christmas tree, signed
Hollycraft, 1940

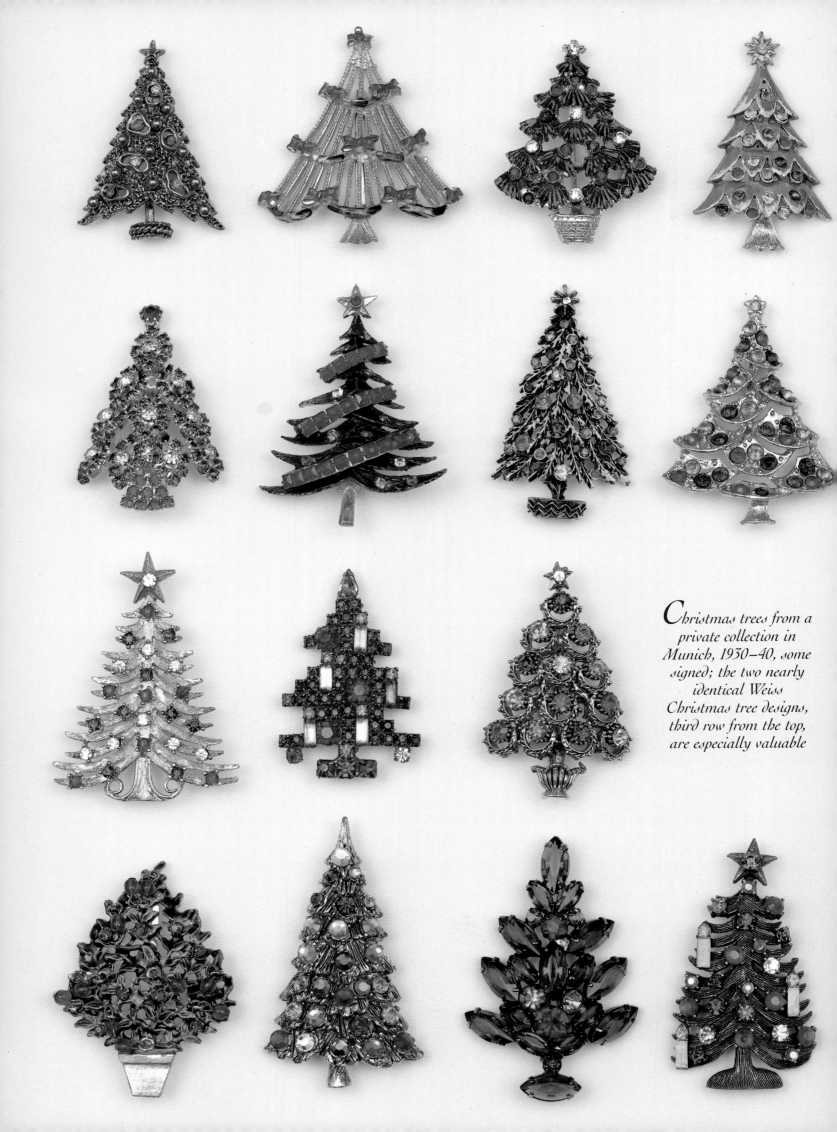

Christmas trees from a private collection in Munich, 1930–40, some signed; the two nearly identical Weiss Christmas tree designs, third row from the top, are especially valuable

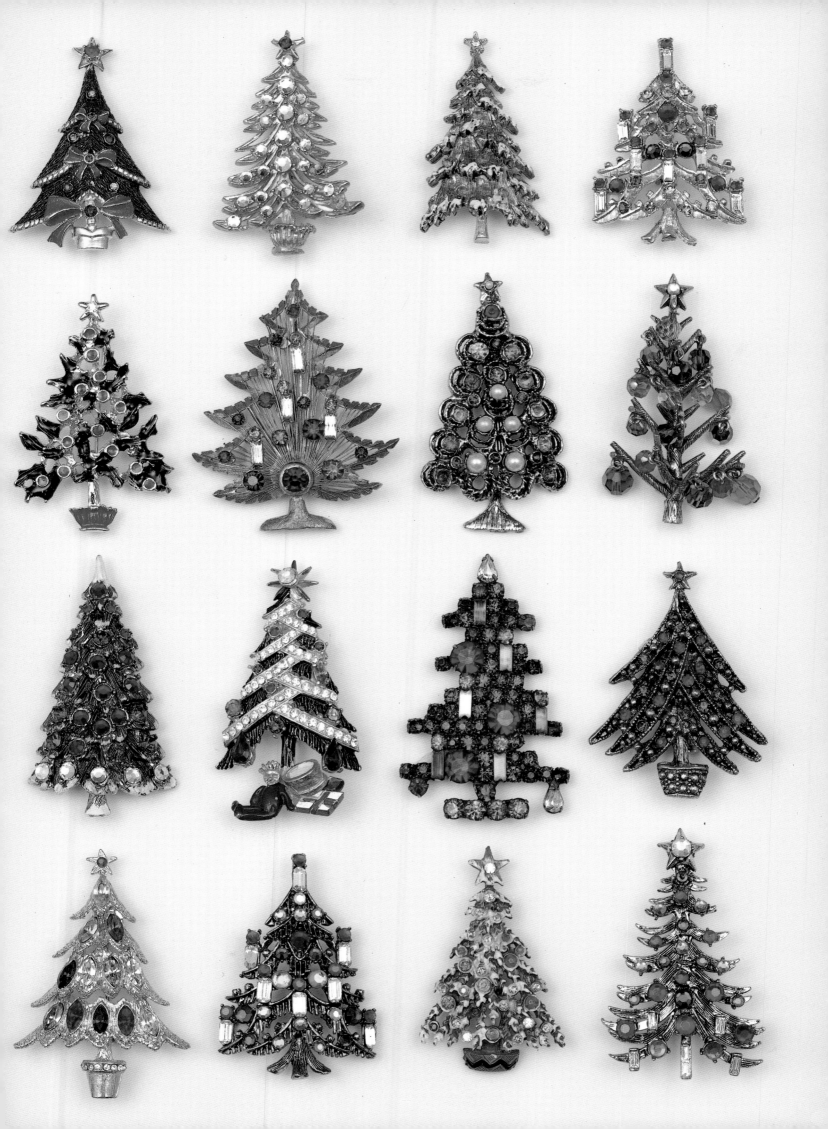

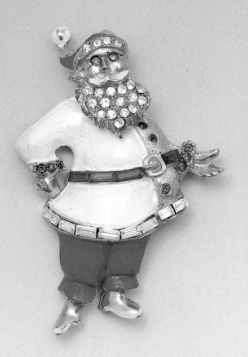
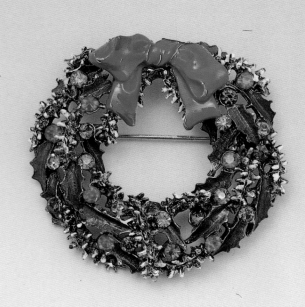

*L*EFT: *Santa Claus, rhinestones and baguette-cut rhinestones and colored metal, 1940*
*R*IGHT: *Christmas wreath pin of holly branches, 1945*

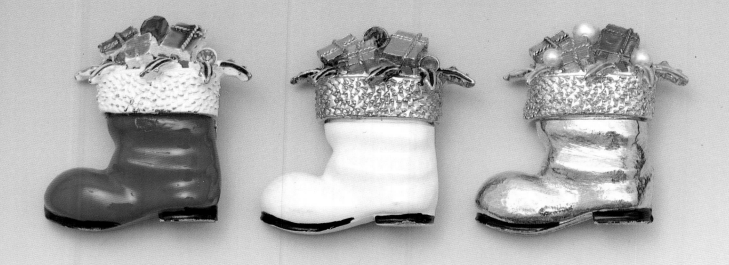

Three Christmas boot pins stuffed with presents; rhinestones, faux pearls, and painted metal, 1940–50

Rhinestones: Collecting and Care

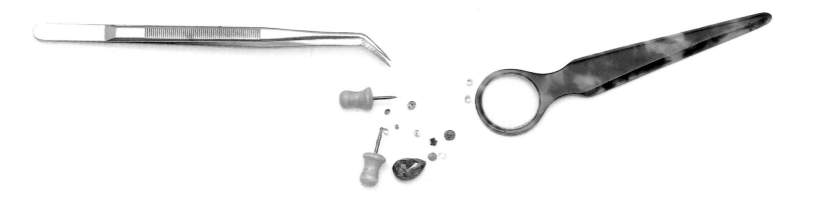

This is certainly the most personal chapter of this book, because like every enthusiast and collector of pretty things, I have my own methods of care and favorite places to search for antique rhinestone brooches, earrings, bracelets, and necklaces.

The collecting of antique rhinestone pieces has become a real passion for many people today, not just for fashion-conscious women. A good ten years ago, when I began to buy these pretty, glittering artworks at flea markets, I was still able to find the oldest pieces — shoe buckles from the eighteenth century, for example — for five or ten dollars. And I began to collect without knowing much about the jewelry, and even less about Georges Frédéric Stras and the history of rhinestone jewelry. I was fascinated with their beauty and craftsmanship and I was enthused about the trick of sprucing up plain blouses with old brooches or wearing a shoe buckle on a satin band as a necklace.

The treatments of antique jewelry — the settings surrounding every single stone, the filigree back of rhinestone brooches from the turn of the century — were worthy of attention on the basis of their perfect craftsmanship. Some of the very old pieces from the eighteenth century are truly unusual, from the lead glass used for the rhinestones to the old cuts of the stones and their settings.

That these old, precious pieces are available almost exclusively at big auctions these days is further indication that the collectors' market for rhinestone jewelry has grown considerably. For over two years one of the leading English auction houses has regularly held auctions of designer costume jewelry. Even though these auctions are not held at the headquarters in London but in a small annex on the outskirts of the city, the very fact that they take place at all shows that the interest of the public is increasing.

It has long been possible to find pretty rhinestone jewelry in various antique shops and at flea markets. The prices in antique stores tend to be somewhat higher, as is generally the case with such dealers. With a relatively new collectors' object such as rhinestone jewelry, an overview of the market is very useful, because private advertisements for antique rhinestone jewelry appear again and again. These private sales frequently pre-sent good opportunities. Of course, careful attention should be paid to the condition of the jewelry being offered for sale: has it been cleaned properly, are any stones missing or scratched, and, naturally, does a designer's signature appear on the item?

In the United States rhinestone jewelry has been methodically collected for the last twenty years and extensive collections have been assembled, some of which specialize in certain jewelry types or styles. Found at flea markets, garage sales, and in small shops, the prettiest rhinestone objects always bring high prices. Signed pieces, especially those made by Trifari, Coro, Hobé, Bogoff, and above all, the wonderful brooches and clips by Eisenberg that are identified as "Eisenberg Original" and date from before 1942, have received and still do receive the highest prices. Some ten years ago an Eisenberg Original might have sold for two hundred dollars, but today it would sell for much more — provided such a rarity is to be found for sale at all.

And this certainly is one of the primary problems all collectors experience. Exquisite pieces, such as the large colored Eisenberg flowers, rarely turn up on the market anymore. Of course, they change ownership time and again at major auctions, but it isn't hard to imagine what kind of price they will command. When Christie's announced the first international auction for costume and rhinestone jewelry to be held in 1989 in London, all its catalogs were swept up in no time and prices for the precious, rare, signed pieces skyrocketed.

Meanwhile, in Europe and elsewhere it is not at all unusual for successful jewelers to showcase antique rhinestone jewelry for sale. Decorative and carefully crafted Art Deco works, especially signed pieces, are already being traded for higher prices. Distinctive rarities, such as a Bogoff chain, and the rarest pieces of all, such as Eisenberg Original clips and brooches, are virtually priceless. Even so, one occasionally has the great luck to discover one of these treasures for sale at a halfway agreeable price. One must only search patiently and be informed.

Some caution, however, is recommended: an object may be a completely legitimate copy with no signature or with only the signature of the modern manufacturer, or it may be an imitation deliberately intended to deceive the customer.

Should one have the luck to find an old piece of rhinestone jewelry at a flea market or a collectors' fair, it must first be cleaned of any dirt accumulated from its wearing and storage. There are many ways to go about this.

Many collectors swear by the use of lukewarm water to clean their jewelry. Dirt and dust is simply and gently washed away with soapsuds. Most who use this cleaning method are aware that some of the old stones may fall out of their settings in the process. For this reason one should never clean the jewelry directly under running water, but in a small basin. The jewelry should be gone over carefully with a soft brush. Only when it is certain that no more stones will fall out can the rest of the soapsuds be rinsed off under cold running water.

The cleaned jewelry is then laid on a cloth towel to dry. Should there be some dirt remaining, the brush and soap can of course be used once again or — in especially stubborn cases — a jeweler's ultrasonic cleaner may be used.

Some collectors, however, never let water touch their jewelry pieces. Their concern is valid to some extent, because the foliation of each individual rhinestone is very fragile indeed. In my completely subjective experience, careful cleaning using soapsuds has never distressed the foliation.

Stronger detergents such as glass cleaner can also be employed if used with caution and very sparingly. Poured into a basin into which a soft brush or cotton swab can be dipped to clean the individual stones, this solvent can bring out a radiant sparkle.

With very old pieces set into silver the first question one should ask is whether it is desirable to remove the patina that gives the jewelry a touch of nostalgia. Should the gleam be re-

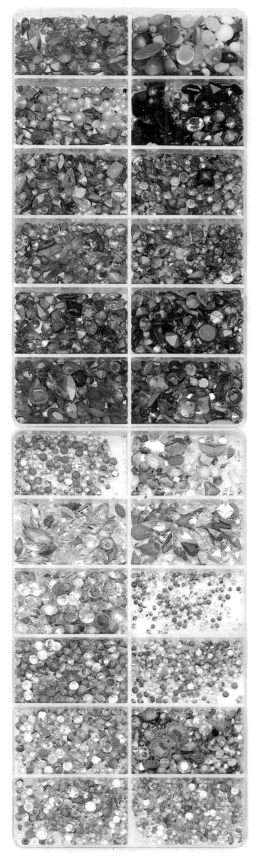

stored to the silver with careful application of a silver polish? Personally, I have never done this, because for me the individual patina contributes to the fascination of a piece of jewelry. The stones in such pieces can be carefully cleaned to restore their glitter, while the silver can be left with its traces of oxidation.

Even with all the care in the world, individual stones are bound to loosen in the process of cleaning. Replacement of the loose stones after cleaning requires a very steady hand. In order to work with precision a loupe should be used. Working with tweezers or fingers, whichever is more sensible considering the size of the stone, one should first clearly establish which stones belong where. Once this has been ascertained, a suitable glue can be applied into the depression with a needle or a small pin and the stone can be reset.

The same procedure applies when a defective piece is purchased at a low price. It is always worth the effort with signed designer jewelry, because a pretty jewelry piece lacking one or two stones can be gotten for very little and — with the necessary patience — is easily repaired. New rhinestones can be purchased in hobby or craft shops and in certain jewelry stores. New stones, however, often differ from the old in color and brilliance. But, with some perseverance, one can find stones of suitably good quality to replace the missing ones in old jewelry. And yet in some cases it is not possible to substitute a new rhinestone in a piece that contains only old stones because even colorless stones can be very different in their refractive quality. The more practiced the eye, the more noticeable the difference seems. Seasoned collectors always buy old, broken-up jewelry pieces, remove the

An assortment of white and colored rhinestones for restoring old pieces

stones, and keep them to replace missing stones in valuable jewelry.

There are almost as many ideas on how to preserve expensive rhinestone jewelry as there are collectors. Many enthusiasts store their treasures nestled in black or blue velvet pockets, others store each individual piece in a separate small pouch, and still others decorate their apartments with them. Jewelry cases or picture frames hung on walls can be very useful for creating ever-changing private home exhibitions.

One thing is true for every method of storage: the rhinestone pieces should never simply be laid next to one another because they can scrape against one another and become damaged.

Scratched stones or foliations not only lower the value of the piece but destroy the visual effect. Old pieces, especially those in which the foliation was as yet unprotected, are often damaged enough and certainly should not be damaged further by careless handling.

Should one have the great fortune to buy a pair of earrings in their original box, this is not only the best means of storing the earrings but another collector's item as well. But the instances of finding old rhinestone jewelry still in its original box are extraordinarily rare. In the years after the war these boxes were made of simple cardboard, on which the manufacturer and the name of the jewelry piece were printed. Still, with the packaging or without, the jewelry itself will always delight its owner.

A completely different problem arises with the wearing of rare pieces: security. Considering the value of such jewelry today, no one would simply put on an Eisenberg Original fur clasp with nothing but the original fastener — two pins that were merely pushed into the fur — the danger of loss would be too great. Some resourceful collectors make a loop out of silver handicraft wire and fasten it between the two pins to give their fur clasps greater security.

A jeweler specializing in safety fastenings can, of course, also give advice in this area. In the past many women simply had the old pins or clips taken off and new, more secure fasteners put on. One of my favorite pieces is just such a "mangled" Eisenberg. Of a wonderful topaz brown, this clip was remounted decades ago. While that has reduced its value today, it most certainly has done no damage to its beauty.

OPPOSITE: Signatures and hallmarks on the undersides of various pieces of rhinestone jewelry containing pure silver
TOP: signed Eisenberg Original
CENTER, FROM LEFT TO RIGHT: signed Eisenberg Ice, Trifari, Weiss
BOTTOM, FROM LEFT TO RIGHT: sterling silver hallmark ensuring that the content of pure silver is 92.5 percent; silver triangle bears sterling hallmark and signature of the manufacturer, Hobé; signature Coro Duette

Signatures

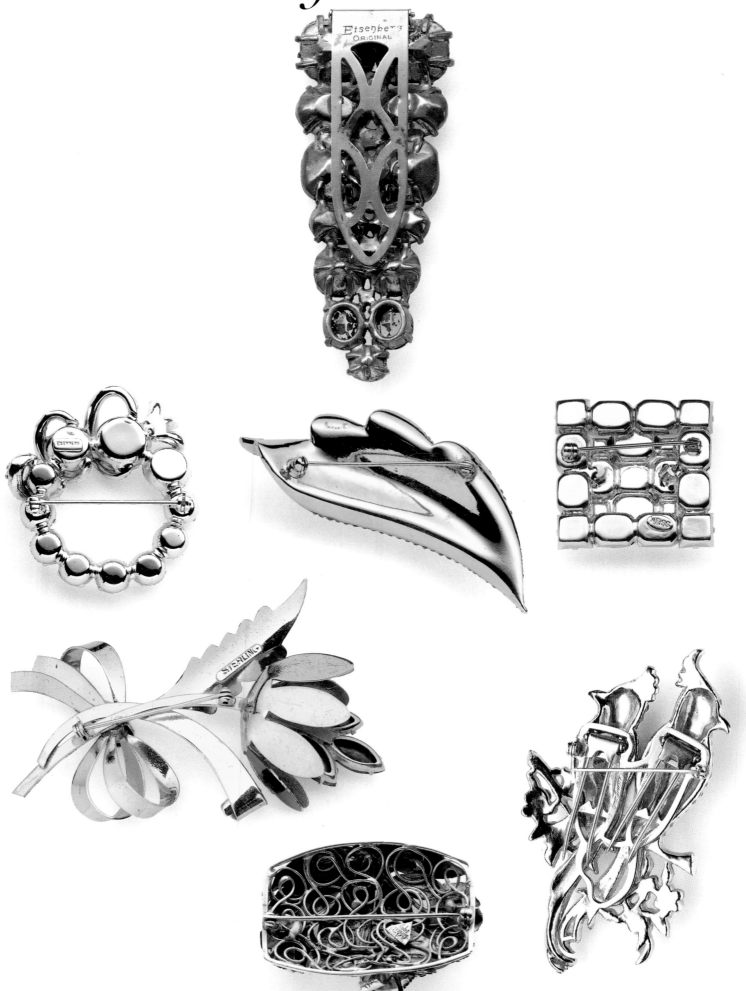

Acknowledgments

We would like to thank all those who have supported this book.

The long and varied work of all those directly involved has directly contributed to the success of this book as well — the first, in our opinion, to place rhinestone jewelry in its proper light — such as the generous support of the collectors whose private collections we searched to photograph pieces.

First among them to be thanked is Mrs. Mary Sue Packer, of Munich and Memphis, Tennessee. We are no less indebted to the Honorable Nick and Linda Tollemache, of Beverly Hills, California, who without hesitation placed the fine pieces from their collection at our disposal. This collection was further supplemented with the collections of Frau Hannelore Riegel, of Munich, Frau Roswitha Heyne, and the author.

Museums and Collections

*B*ecause rhinestone jewelry has until now received consideration only as a highly specialized field of art history, there exists as yet no international catalog of all the large and small museums that have collections of this jewelry.

Thus, the following listing of museums, collections, and exhibitions is only an overview, gathered on the basis of personal familiarity and the available literature.

It should also be noted that in most museums costume jewelry is presented in the decorative arts department, and a few museums, such as the Johanneum in Graz, Austria, are increasingly giving greater attention to costume jewelry — rhinestone jewelry in particular — and to a scholarly assessment of it as well.

Boston, Society for Preservation of New England Antiquities
Dearborn, Michigan, Henry Ford Museum
Frankfurt, Museum für Kunsthandwerk
Glasgow, Art Gallery and Museum
Graz, Austria, Johanneum, Abteilung für Kunstgewerbe
Kaufbeuren, Germany, Schmuckmuseum Neugablonz
Kenwood, England, Lady Maufe Collection
London, British Museum
London, Victoria and Albert Museum
Milan, Pellini Collection
New York, The Brooklyn Museum
New York, Cooper-Hewitt Museum
New York, Napier
Nuremberg, Gewerbemuseum der Landesgewerbeanstalt im Germanischen Nationalmuseum
Paris, Musée des Arts Décoratifs
Pforzheim, Germany, Schmuckmuseum
Vienna, Österreichisches Museum für angewandte Kunst
Washington, D.C., Division of Costume, National Museum of American History

Selected Bibliography

Baker, Lillian. *Fifty Years of Collectible Fashion, Jewelry, 1925–1975.* Paducah, Ky., 1986.
Becker, Vivienne. *Fabulous Fakes: The History of Fantasy and Fashion Jewellery.* London, 1988.
Black, J. Anderson. *The Story of Jewelry.* New York, 1974.
Bott, Gerhard. *Ullstein Juwelenbuch.* Berlin, Frankfurt am Main, and Vienna, 1972.
Bury, Shirley. *An Introduction to Sentimental Jewellery.* Owings Mills, Md., 1985.
Buxbaum, Gerda. *Mode aus Wien, 1815–1938.* Salzburg, Vienna, 1986.
Charles-Roux, Edmonde. *Le temps Chanel.* Paris, 1979.

Dolan, Maryanne. *Collecting Rhinestone Jewelry: An Identification and Value Guide.* Florence, Ala., 1984.
Egger, Gerhart. *Bürgerlicher Schmuck: 15. bis 20. Jahrhundert.* Munich, 1984.
Ellman, Barbara. *The World of Fashion Jewelry.* Highland Park, Ill., 1986.
Greindl, Gabriele. "Les diamants de Stras: Georges Frédéric Stras (1701–1773) und der Strassschmuck." *Weltkunst* 23 (1988): 3631–35.
Gregorietti, Guido. *Gold und Juwelen: Eine Geschichte des Schmucks von Ur bis Tiffany.* Munich, 1971.
Hase, Ulrike von. *Schmuck in Deutschland und Österreich, 1895–1914: Symbolismus, Jugendstil, Neohistorismus.* Munich, 1977.
Heller, Carl Benno, Ina Schneider, and Walter Dennert, eds. *Bruckmanns Handbuch des Schmucks.* Munich, 1977.
Kamer, Martin. "Brilliant Adornments." In *Revolution in Fashion: European Clothing, 1715–1815,* edited by the Kyoto Costume Institute. New York, 1989.
Kelley, Lyngerda, and Nancy Schiffer. *The Great Pretenders: Costume Jewelry.* West Chester, Pa., 1987.
Kurzel-Runtschneider, Erich. *Pierres de Stras und die Strasser Legende.* Vienna, 1948.
Marquardt, Brigitte. *Schmuck-Klassizismus und Biedermeier 1780–1850: Deutschland, Österreich, Schweiz.* Munich, 1983.
Mulvagh, Jane. *Costume Jewelry in Vogue.* New York, 1988.
Poynder, Michael. *The Price Guide to Jewellery, 3000 B.C.–1950 A.D.* Ithaca, N.Y., 1985.
Raulet, Sylvie. *Schmuck Art Déco.* Munich, 1985.
———. *Schmuck der vierziger und fünfziger Jahre.* Munich, 1987.
Rössler, Susanne. *Gablonzer Glas und Schmuck: Tradition und Gegenwart einer kunsthandlichen Industrie.* Munich, 1979.
Rothmüller, Hans. *Schmuck und Juwelen: Battenberg Antiquitätenkataloge.* Munich, 1985.
Rücklin, Rudolf. *Das Schmuckbuch,* vol. 2. Leipzig, 1901. Reprint. Hannover, 1982.
Scarisbrick, Diana. *Jewellery.* Costume Accessories Series. London, 1984.
Schiffer, Nancy N. *Costume Jewelry: The Fun of Collecting.* West Chester, Pa., 1988.
Schmuckmuseum Pforzehim. Braunschweig, Germany, 1981.
Steingräber, Erich. *Alter Schmuck: Die Kunst des europäischen Schmuckes.* Munich, 1956.
Thiel, Erika. *Geschichte des Kostüms: Die europäische Mode von den Anfängen bis zur Gegenwart,* 7th ed. Wilhelmshaven, Germany, 1987.
Trott zu Solz, Petra von. *Stras: Simili-Diamantenschmuck des 18. Jahrhunderts.* Cologne, 1982.
Wermusch, Günter. *Adamas: Diamanten in Geschichte und Geschichten.* Berlin, 1984.
White, Palmer. *Elsa Schiaparelli: Empress of Paris Fashion.* London, 1986.
Zitte, Rudolf. *Die Geschichte der Gablonzer Schmuckindustrie.* Kaufbeuren and Neugablonz, Germany, 1958.

Index

Photography Credits

Bilderdienst Süddeutscher Verlag, 146; Deutsche Presse-Agentur, Munich, 164, 226; English Heritage, The Iveagh Bequest, Kenwood, 40; Hubs Flöter/Dieter Hinrichs, Munich, 180; Gamma, Paris, 152; Archive Dr. Karkosch, Gilching near Munich, 84, 128, 142, 200; The Kobal Collection, London, 66, 76, 106, 174, 206; Studio X, Paris, 44; Trifari, New York, 192; Gianni Versace, Milan, 218.